TREATING SLEEP PROBLEMS

Treating
Sleep Problems

A TRANSDIAGNOSTIC APPROACH

Allison G. Harvey
Daniel J. Buysse

THE GUILFORD PRESS
New York   London

Printed in the United States of America

This book is printed on acid-free paper.

Last digit is print number: 9   8   7   6   5   4   3   2   1

The authors have checked with sources believed to be reliable in their efforts to provide
information that is complete and generally in accord with the standards of practice
that are accepted at the time of publication. However, in view of the possibility of
human error or changes in behavioral, mental health, or medical sciences, neither the
authors, nor the editors and publisher, nor any other party who has been involved in
the preparation or publication of this work warrants that the information contained
herein is in every respect accurate or complete, and they are not responsible for any
errors or omissions or the results obtained from the use of such information. Readers are
encouraged to confirm the information contained in this book with other sources.

Library of Congress Cataloging-in-Publication Data

Names: Harvey, Allison G., 1968– author. | Buysse, Daniel J., author.
Title: Treating sleep problems : a transdiagnostic approach / Allison G.
    Harvey, Daniel J. Buysse.
Description: New York : The Guilford Press, [2017] | Includes bibliographical
    references and index.
Identifiers: LCCN 2017024443| ISBN 9781462531950 (paperback : alk. paper) |
    ISBN 9781462531967 (hardcover : alk. paper)
Subjects: | MESH: Sleep Initiation and Maintenance Disorders—therapy |
    Chronobiology Disorders—therapy | Cognitive Therapy—methods
Classification: LCC RC548 | NLM WM 188 | DDC 616.8/4982—dc23
LC record available at https://lccn.loc.gov/2017024443

To my mentors, Richard A. Bryant, David M. Clark, Anke Ehlers,
Christopher G. Fairburn, Ronald M. Rapee, and Paul M. Salkovskis,
who are extraordinarily creative and inspiring clinical scientists

And to my husband, Henry Hieslmair, and our soon-to-be-born son,
who has kept me company with his sweet fluttering
and gentle kicks as this book was written

—A. G. H.

To my mentors, David J. Kupfer, Charles F. Reynolds III,
and Timothy H. Monk,
who taught me not only about sleep, rhythms, and science,
but also about the importance of mentoring itself—I stand on your shoulders

—D. J. B.

About the Authors

Allison G. Harvey, PhD, is Professor of Psychology at the University of California, Berkeley, where she is Director of the Golden Bear Sleep and Mood Research Clinic. Dr. Harvey has practiced as a cognitive-behavioral therapist since the 1990s, specializing in sleep problems, and has published over 250 peer-reviewed articles and chapters. She is the recipient of numerous awards, including the President's New Research Award from the Association for Behavioral and Cognitive Therapies, the Beck Scholar Award for Excellence in Contributions to Cognitive Therapy from the Beck Institute for Cognitive Behavior Therapy, the Young Investigator Award from the Brain and Behavior Research Foundation, and an honorary doctorate from the University of Orebro, Sweden. She is a Fellow of the Association for Psychological Science.

Daniel J. Buysse, MD, is the UPMC Professor of Sleep Medicine and Professor of Psychiatry and Clinical and Translational Science at the University of Pittsburgh. His research focuses on sleep assessment, the pathophysiology and treatment of insomnia, interactions between sleep and circadian rhythms, and the impact of sleep on health. Dr. Buysse has published over 300 peer-reviewed articles and over 100 book chapters or review articles. He is past president of the American Academy of Sleep Medicine, a recipient of the Mary A. Carskadon Outstanding Educator Award from the Sleep Research Society, and Deputy Editor of the journal *SLEEP*.

Preface

We have both spent our careers with a primary clinical and research interest in insomnia. However, as we sought to treat a broad range of youth and adults with sleep problems, we noticed that in many cases insomnia was not the only sleep problem that people were experiencing. Moreover, as we surveyed the research literature and conducted our own research, the complexity of sleep problems was also clearly apparent. For example, insomnia often overlaps with features of circadian rhythm disorders, such as delayed sleep phase and irregular sleep–wake schedules. Yet we also noticed that the majority of studies within the sleep field are focused on disorders—that is, they tend to treat a specific sleep problem, typically insomnia. Moreover, the existing disorder-focused research provided few clinical guidelines on how to treat the more complex clients. This core observation was one factor that motivated us to develop the Transdiagnostic Sleep and Circadian Intervention (TranS-C).

Another motivating factor came from the burgeoning literature on sleep disturbances as risk factors for adverse health outcomes. It has now been well established that both short and long sleep duration are associated with such risks, but newer literature has also shown that sleep timing, daytime napping or sleepiness, sleep quality, sleep efficiency, and sleep regularity pose risks of their own. While it may make sense to consider these various dimensions *individually* for scientific purposes, the reality is that they occur *simultaneously* among people living in the real world. Thus, from a scientific as well as a clinical perspective, the time has come to wrestle with sleep as the complex, multidimensional phenomenon it really is.

Our formal collaboration began in 2008, when we submitted a grant application to the National Institute of Mental Health as an initial test of the transdiagnostic, multidimensional perspective among individuals who met diagnostic criteria for bipolar disorder as well as insomnia. In this study we decided to *not* exclude the many participants who presented with insomnia and clinical features of hypersomnia, delayed sleep phase, and other such comorbid sleep problems. We selected bipolar disorder for this first study for three reasons. First, sleep and circadian disturbances are prominent features of bipolar disorder. Second, the empirical evidence indicates that sleep and circadian disturbance may be one causal pathway that leads to relapse in bipolar disorder. Third, sleep and circadian disturbance in bipolar disorder is complicated and often includes features of insomnia, delayed sleep phase, hypersomnia, and irregular sleep–wake schedules. Hence, an approach that treats this broader range of sleep problems seemed warranted. We scoured the scientific literature to obtain guidance on how to target these complicated features of sleep in bipolar disorder. In line with the treatment development method proposed by Onken, Carroll, Shoham, Cuthbert, and Riddle (2014), we realized that we may be able to target several of these important features of the sleep problems experienced by people with bipolar disorder by supplementing cognitive-behavioral therapy for insomnia (CBT-I) with elements from three existing evidence-based treatments: interpersonal and social rhythm therapy (IPSRT; Frank, 2005; Frank et al., 2005), chronotherapy (Wirz-Justice, Benedetti, & Terman, 2009), and motivational interviewing (MI; Miller & Rollnick, 2013). These therapies provided the groundwork for a new approach that formed the basis for TranS-C. Our initial test of the new intervention improved sleep and mood outcomes in individuals diagnosed with bipolar disorder (Harvey et al., 2015).

Over the past few years, we have also been developing a new theoretical perspective on sleep that complements our clinical experiences and influenced the development of TranS-C. The "sleep health" framework (Buysse, 2014) begins with the recognition that sleep is an important pathway to overall health. However, leveraging sleep to maximize health involves much more than identifying and treating sleep and circadian disorders—the traditional sleep medicine perspective. The sleep health framework adopts a health promotion perspective, in which we endeavour to facilitate each client truly becoming a "good sleeper." The sleep health framework focuses on six dimensions of sleep: Regularity, referring to going to sleep at about the same time each night and waking up at about the same time each morning; Satisfaction with sleep or sleep quality, referring to the subjective assessment of "good" or "poor" sleep made by the patient; Alertness during waking hours or daytime sleepiness, focusing on the patient's ability to maintain attentive wakefulness during the daytime; Timing, which refers to the placement of the patient's sleep within the

24-hour day; sleep **E**fficiency, referring to the ability to sleep for a large percentage of the time in bed, as indicated by the ease of falling asleep at the beginning of the night and the ease of returning to sleep after awakenings during the night; and sleep **D**uration, which refers to the total amount of sleep obtained every 24 hours. Note the acronym RU SATED here! The goal of TranS-C is to encourage optimal sleep across each of these six dimensions.

Another key motivator for us both has been the recognition of a critical problem in the mental health field. In most countries, mental health professionals are concentrated in highly populated, relatively affluent urban areas. Yet the millions of people with a mental disorder are geographically distributed, and live in low-income and rural areas as well. Unfortunately, this dearth of local providers is an international problem (Kazdin & Blase, 2011; Kazdin & Rabbitt, 2013). Then consider the likely group of people who would benefit from a sleep treatment—a huge number—as we discuss in Chapter 1. Consider also that among the mental health professionals available, only a handful have the background to confidently treat sleep problems. (In a recent survey of clinical psychology programs, only 6% offered a course in sleep problems and only 31% offered training in sleep treatment [Meltzer, Phillips, & Mindell, 2009].) The high prevalence of sleep problems, together with the paucity of treatment providers, indicates a pressing need for continued innovation to improve the transportability and usefulness of current treatments to front-line providers. Thus, a sleep-focused treatment that applies to a *variety of sleep problems* comorbid with a *variety of mental disorders*, and that can be used confidently by a *variety of mental health professionals*, provides yet another motivation for TranS-C. Also, a treatment such as TranS-C is more scalable nationally and internationally relative to multiple disorder-focused treatments, such as cognitive-behavioral therapy for delayed phase in depression (CBT-DP-D), CBT-I for insomnia in schizophrenia (CBT-I-S), and so on.

The TranS-C intervention has been informed by several treatment development traditions. First, *psychosocial treatments* often emerge through a consensus between skilled clinician-researchers. Many *medication treatments* have been discovered by serendipity or by modifying or copying other effective drugs (although an increased understanding of the mechanisms of diseases is beginning to lead to more targeted drug discovery). Perhaps not surprisingly, there have been calls for increased attention to science as the optimal pathway toward more highly efficient and effective treatments (Insel, 2009). Indeed, such methods have been used to develop effective psychosocial treatments with impressive outcomes (Insel, 2009). Following in this tradition, we endeavored to use scientific evidence to support both the *development* and the *content* of each component of TranS-C. Second, Onken et al.'s (2014) stage model of treatment development points out that intervention generation ("Stage 2") can draw from a variety of sources, including basic science ("Stage 1") as well as existing efficacy research ("Stage 3"). As described later in this book, TranS-C is derived from both basic science and existing efficacy research. Third, David M. Clark, Anke Ehlers, and Paul Salkovskis (Clark, 1999, 2004; Clark et al., 1999; Ehlers & Clark, 2000; Salkovskis, 2002) emphasize that clinical practice is essential for generating hypotheses about where further innovation and treatment development are needed. This approach also emphasizes that hypotheses generated via clinical practice need to be tested with research, which can then be used to derive a scientifically tested theory about the maintenance of the problem. This theory evolves into a "road map" for developing novel treatments. The treatment techniques that aim to reverse the maintaining processes specified in the theory are also scientifically tested before being combined into a multicomponent approach. This step-by-step approach was critical to the development of TranS-C.

Of course, a final influence on the development of TranS-C has been the broader movement toward transdiagnostic treatments (Barlow, Allen, & Choate, 2004; Fairburn, Cooper, & Shafran, 2003; Harvey, Watkins, Mansell, & Shafran, 2004). Transdiagnostic treatments have been developed for anxiety disorders and depression (Ellard, Fairholme, Boisseau, Farchione, & Barlow, 2010; Norton & Philipp, 2008; Titov et al., 2011); eating disorders (Fairburn et al., 2009); paranoid delusions (Bentall et al., 2009); bipolar disorder and comorbid anxiety (Ellard et al., 2010); and anxiety, depression, and conduct problems in youth (Weisz et al., 2012). Treatments targeting transdiagnostic processes, such as rumination (Nolen-Hoeksema & Watkins, 2011) and perfectionism (Egan, Wade, & Shafran, 2011), have been effective for a range of different disorders (Riley, Lee, Cooper, Fairburn, & Shafran, 2007; Watkins et al., 2011). We are delighted and excited to add an approach for sleep and circadian problems to this rapidly growing list.

Acknowledgments

We are deeply grateful to our spouses, Henry Hieslmair and Sandra Buysse, for their constant support and encouragement even as we both devote many hours every week to our sleep research in addition to our typical "office hours."

We are endlessly thankful to those individuals who have participated in our research studies and attended our clinics for treatment. Research and clinical care are partnerships. We recognize our patient-participant partners for teaching and guiding us as we honed and developed treatment approaches that will reach the broadest possible range of people experiencing sleep and circadian problems.

We are indebted to the National Institutes of Health (NIH) for support that resulted in, and was essential for crafting, the body of work that resulted in this book (Grant Nos. HD071065, MH079188, MH082034, AG20677, AG047139, MH102412, HL125103, and MH078961). The rigor and quality of the peer review process at NIH has been a critical influence on the direction this work has taken.

Many talented, rigorous, and inspiring clinician-researchers have each influenced this approach for more than 20 years, including David M. Clark, David J. Kupfer, Christopher G. Fairburn, Ellen Frank, Joel Sherrill, Eve Fine, Kerry Kulstad-Thomas, Melissa J. Ree, Gregory N. Clarke, Charles M. Morin, Ronald E. Dahl, Charles F. Reynolds, Dana L. McMakin, Kerrie Hein, Rita Smith, Monique Thompson, Kate Kaplan, Deidre Abrons, Hanna Mark, Mike Dolsen, Niki Gumport, Caitlin Eggleston, Lulu Dong, Laurie Brar, Mark Jones, Stephen P. Hinshaw, Emily J. Ozer, Daniel Freeman, Jorin Bukosky, and Donna

E. Rinaldo. We are grateful to each and every one of them for discussions and supervision sessions that have encouraged us to keep focused on the issues that matter by embracing scientific rigor while retaining compassion and creativity.

Finally, we are grateful to Jim Nageotte, Senior Editor, Barbara Watkins, Developmental Editor, Jane Keislar, Senior Assistant Editor, and Jeannie Tang, Senior Production Editor, from The Guilford Press. Their feedback, guidance, and help throughout the process of developing this book has been greatly appreciated.

Contents

Purchasers of this book can download and print enlarged versions of select materials at *www.guilford.com/harvey3-forms* for personal use or use with clients (see copyright page for details).

CHAPTER 1

Promoting Healthy Sleep

Sleep is that golden chain that ties health
and our bodies together.
—THOMAS DEKKER (1572–1632)

The Goodness of Sleep

Over the past 5 decades an avalanche of discoveries has documented the benefits of healthy sleep and the functioning of the 24-hour (circadian) clock. Healthy sleep and circadian functioning improve every aspect of our lives. Emotionally we are better regulated, happier, and less prone to developing mental illness. Cognitively we are more attentive, learn more effectively, remember more completely, and think more creatively. Physically we regulate our body weight more easily, increase our activity level, clear toxic brain molecules more thoroughly, and show improved immune system functioning. Healthy sleep and circadian rhythms are associated with a lower incidence of depression, Alzheimer's disease, diabetes, cardiovascular disease, and even of the common cold. A good night's sleep allows us to stay alert and function well at work and in our social and family lives, and to remain more motivated and more likely to achieve our personal goals. It also helps with daily routines, such as driving more safely. Finally, healthy sleep and circadian functioning are linked to reduced mortality risk—meaning that good sleepers live better *and* longer lives. Clearly, there are compelling reasons to place a high priority on establishing healthy sleep and circadian function patterns. Promoting optimal sleep health is an often-overlooked pathway toward optimizing mental and physical health.

The Sleep Health Framework

The goal of this book is to describe a novel treatment approach, the Transdi-agnostic Sleep and Circadian Intervention (TranS-C), which we propose as a pathway to promote *sleep health*. The sleep health framework (Buysse, 2014) underlies and guides TranS-C. Within this framework, the pathway to improv-ing sleep health involves identifying and treating sleep disorders, such as insom-nia, and circadian rhythm disorders, such as advanced or delayed sleep-phase problems. There is robust evidence showing that these disorders are associ-ated with a broad range of negative emotional and health outcomes. However, the sleep health framework encourages us to go much further. Indeed, healthy sleep and circadian functioning is much more than the absence of sleep disor-ders. The goal of promoting sleep health is to optimize clients' ability to truly become "good sleepers."

The sleep health framework represents a shift from the typical sleep medicine perspective, which emphasizes the identification and treatment of sleep disorders, to a *health promotion* perspective, which emphasizes universal attributes of sleep that can be optimized to promote well-being. The approach is informed by four perspectives on sleep and health: (1) the *medical model*, which emphasizes the treatment of sleep disorders; (2) the approach taken by the World Health Organization, which encompasses *health and well-being* in physical, mental, and social domains; (3) *wellness* and role performance models, which encourage the integration of body, mind, and spirit; and (4) models that incorporate the importance of an individual being able to adapt to challenges in the physical and social *environment*. Based on these perspectives, we propose the following definition of sleep health:

> Sleep health is a multidimensional pattern of sleep-wakefulness, adapted to individual, social, and environmental demands, that promotes physical and mental well-being. Good sleep health is characterized by subjective satisfac-tion, appropriate timing, adequate duration, high efficiency, and sustained alertness during waking hours. (Buysse, 2014, p. 12)

More recent research has also led us to emphasize the regularity of sleep–wake patterns since regularity in itself is associated with better health out-comes. Thus, the framework encourages clinicians to work toward improving client's sleep along six dimensions:

- Dimension 1: <u>R</u>egularity. This dimension refers to going to sleep and waking up at about the same times.
- Dimension 2: <u>S</u>atisfaction with sleep or sleep quality. This dimension

refers to the subjective assessment of "good" or "poor" sleep made by the client.

- Dimension 3: <u>A</u>lertness during waking hours. This dimension is focused on the client's ability to maintain attentive wakefulness during the daytime and not to experience unwanted daytime sleepiness.
- Dimension 4: <u>T</u>iming. This dimension refers to the placement of the client's sleep within the 24-hour day.
- Dimension 5: Sleep <u>E</u>fficiency. This dimension refers to the ability to sleep for a large percentage of the time in bed, as indicated by the ease of falling asleep at the beginning of the night and the ease of returning to sleep after awakenings during the night.
- Dimension 6: Sleep <u>D</u>uration. This dimension refers to the total amount of sleep obtained by the client over 24 hours.

These dimensions can be easily remembered with the relevant acronym RU SATED—that is, has your sleep "filled up" your emotional, cognitive, and physical need to sleep? These dimensions can be assessed on a continuum and for four of them, a *higher score is better.* However, for dimensions 4 and 6, sleep timing and healthy sleep duration, we seek a middle road. Sleep duration that is either too long or too short and sleep timing that is too early or too late may be associated with negative health outcomes. All of these dimensions can be quantified by self-report measures, such as the retrospective questionnaires and sleep diary discussed in Chapter 2. These dimensions can also be measured behaviorally (actigraphy) and physiologically (polysomnography). However, actigraphy and polysomnography are not often required in clinical practice. Finally, there is a sound empirical basis for each of the six dimensions as reviewed in detail in Buysse (2014) and briefly described here.

- *Regularity* in sleep and wake times is a relatively new focus of research (Bei, Wiley, Trinder, & Manber, 2016). Irregularity has already been associated with poor school performance, insomnia, bipolar disorder, circadian rhythm disorders, negative health outcomes, and obesity.
- *Satisfaction with sleep.* Lack of sleep satisfaction, a hallmark of insomnia, is associated with metabolic syndrome, diabetes, hypertension, coronary heart disease, and depression.
- *Alertness during waking hours.* The opposite of alertness, daytime sleepiness, is associated with increased mortality risk, coronary heart disease, and impaired neurobehavioral performance.
- *Timing of sleep.* Research done on shift work and "chronotype"—our preference for early or late bedtimes—has found that sleep taken at very

early or very late times is associated with increased mortality risk, coronary heart disease, metabolic syndrome, diabetes, and accidents.

* *Sleep efficiency.* Poor sleep efficiency has been associated with increased mortality risk, coronary heart disease, metabolic syndrome, hypertension, and depression.

* *Sleep duration* that is too short or too long has been associated with mortality, obesity, metabolic syndrome, diabetes, hypertension, coronary heart disease, and impaired neurobehavioral performance.

Around 20% of adults in the general population meet the criteria for insomnia. Comorbidity between psychiatric disorders and insomnia is estimated to fall between 41 and 53% (e.g., Benca, Obermeyer, Thisted, & Gillin, 1992; Breslau, Roth, Rosenthal, & Andreski, 1996; Buysse et al., 1994; Ford & Kamerow, 1989). If the estimates for insomnia are combined with the estimates for other common sleep problems, such as delayed and advanced sleep phase disorder and hypersomnia (e.g., Gradisar, Gardner, & Dohnt, 2011; Liu et al., 2007), a large segment of the population is affected, with high personal and societal costs (Daley, Morin, LeBlanc, Gregoire, & Savard, 2009; Hillman, Murphy, & Pezzullo, 2006; Ozminkowski, Wang, & Walsh, 2007; Roth et al., 2006). If we add another large segment of the population who don't meet formal diagnostic criteria for a sleep disorder but who fall short on one or more of the six dimensions of sleep health to this group, then clearly there are a huge number of people who would benefit from a sleep treatment.

To summarize, TranS-C aims to go beyond ameliorating categorically defined sleep and circadian disorders to facilitating clients' ability to achieve the definition of good sleep health offered earlier. The goal of TranS-C is to help the client optimize each of the six sleep health dimensions.

Key Principles of TranS-C

A Transdiagnostic Approach

At the core of TranS-C is a relatively new approach, namely, targeting research and treatment at "transdiagnostic processes," which are defined as clinical features that are common to more than one mental illness (Barlow, Allen, & Choate, 2004; Fairburn, Cooper, & Shafran, 2003; Harvey, Watkins, Mansell, & Shafran, 2004).

Sleep and circadian dysfunction is a biologically (Harvey, Murray, Chandler, & Soehner, 2011) and theoretically (Harvey, 2008) plausible *transdiagnostic* contributor to mental illness. Indeed, sleep and circadian problems not only coexist with mental disorders but mounting scientific evidence indicates that sleep and circadian problems are important causal or mecha-nistic contributors to mental disorders (e.g., Harvey, 2008). Also, the majority of studies within the sleep field are disorder focused—that is, they tend to treat a specific sleep problem (e.g., insomnia). In contrast, real life sleep and circadian problems are not so neatly categorized. Indeed, insomnia can overlap with features of hypersomnia (Kaplan & Harvey, 2009) and circadian rhythm disorders, such as delayed sleep phase (Giglio et al., 2010; Sivertsen et al., 2013) and irregular sleep–wake schedules (Gruber et al., 2009).

A systematic review (Taylor & Pruiksma, 2014) and a meta-analysis (Wu, Appleman, Salazar, & Ong, 2015) of research on sleep treatments for a range of mental disorders have been published. As just noted, typically these studies have been disorder focused in that they have treated insomnia using cognitive-behavioral therapy for insomnia (CBT-I) in one mental illness. Interestingly, the review concluded that treating sleep problems occurring in depression, anxiety, and posttraumatic stress disorder improves not just the sleep problem but also the comorbid condition. Moreover, a similar pattern of findings has been reported for schizophrenia (Freeman et al., 2015). Even more strikingly, this pattern of findings is not specific to mental illness. Wu et al. (2015) showed a similar pattern of effects across a range of medical disorders including chronic pain, renal disease, cancer, and fibromyalgia, and even two sleep disorders: periodic limb movement disorder and obstructive sleep apnea. Although the effect size for insomnia treatment in medical disorders was smaller than that for mental disorders, the general principle held true—treating sleep problems improves outcomes for comorbid disorders. In short, there are multiple demon-strations that a time-limited sleep treatment is helpful for people who also have a range of mental and physical illnesses, adding to the likely benefit of treating sleep transdiagnostically.

The transdiagnostic approach has several advantages (Harvey et al., 2004). First, if a transdiagnostic process contributes to the maintenance of symptoms across multiple disorders, then focusing treatment on the transdiag-nostic process may be the most efficient approach. Second, many clients meet the diagnostic criteria for more than one mental illness, and in deciding which disorder to prioritize for treatment perhaps we could target treatment at one or more transdiagnostic processes. Relatedly, one account of comorbidity is that the clinical and biological boundaries among mental disorders may not be so distinct (Brown & Barlow, 1992). Thus, basing diagnosis and treatment on clinical signs and symptoms may be imprecise. Third, clinicians who are challenged with learning multiple disorder-focused protocols face a heavy bur-den. Often these protocols have common theoretical underpinnings and even use similar interventions. As such, the transdiagnostic approach may help to address the "too many empirically supported treatments problem" (Weisz, Ng,

& Bearman, 2014, p. 68). TranS-C provides a robust transdiagnostic treatment *framework* that applies to clients with a wide range of mental disorders. The rationale for TranS-C, along with key features described later in this chapter, is summarized in Box 1.1.

The Two-Process Model of Sleep

One of the most widely cited and heuristically useful theories in the sleep field is the two-process model (Borbely & Wirz-Justice, 1982), which is central to TranS-C. This model describes two basic physiological processes that govern the sleep–wake cycle: a circadian process and a homeostatic process.

The *circadian process* is the unfolding of the sleep and wake rhythm across a 24-hour period. It is driven by the "master clock"—the suprachiasmatic nuclei (SCN), which are located within the hypothalamus of the brain

---

BOX 1.1. TranS-C Rationale and Key Characteristics

- Sleep and circadian problems are common and are often associated with mental and physical disorders.

- Sleep and circadian problems are important causal or mechanistic contributors to mental disorders.

- Sleep and circadian problems can occur even in the absence of a specific sleep disorder.

- There is evidence that behavioral and psychological interventions can be used to improve sleep health across a wide range of disorders.

- Most treatment research and the current treatment approaches are focused on insomnia, yet real-life sleep problems are complex and often include other clinical features, such as hypersomnia, delayed ("owls") or advanced ("larks") sleep timing, and irregular sleep–wake schedules.

- TranS-C is transportable and useful to front-line providers working in a broad range of settings.

- TranS-C is empirically derived and draws from existing evidence-based treatments.

- TranS-C helps solve the "too many empirically supported treatments problem" (Weisz et al., 2014, p. 68).

- TranS-C can be personalized to each client's sleep problems.

- TranS-C is relevant to a range of sleep problems across a range of mental disorders.

(Reppert & Weaver, 2002). The SCN have an internal, or endogenous, rhythm that runs close to 24 hours even in the absence of any time cues from the environment. The process by which the master clock synchronizes to the 24-hour day is called *entrainment*. Entrainment occurs via *zeitgebers*, the German word for "time givers." The primary zeitgeber for the circadian process is the daily alteration of light and dark (Roennebert & Foster, 1997). In other words, our exposure to light and dark during the day and night has a major influence on the circadian rhythm in our SCN. Hence, TranS-C incorporates timed light and dark exposure, as we will discuss in detail later. Circadian rhythms can be measured in almost every physiological function, including hormone rhythms, blood pressure, body temperature—and the propensity for sleep. Moreover, circadian rhythms also govern our cognitive, mental, and emotional processes.

Interestingly, evidence from human and animal studies show that the SCN is entrained not only by light, but by other types of zeitgebers, such as arousal, activity, social time, meals, sleep deprivation, and temperature (Mistlberger, Antle, Glass, & Miller, 2000). Hence, TranS-C includes a focus on regularizing the daily sleep–wake rhythm in these nonphotic cues. Again, we will describe the details of the treatment approach later.

If the circadian process is like a clock, the *homeostatic process* is more like an hourglass. Our brain keeps track of the time elapsed since waking, increasing our drive for sleep the longer we are awake. More specifically, the homeostatic pressure to sleep increases during the time we are awake and dissipates during sleep (Jenni, Achermann, & Carskadon, 2005; Taylor, Jenni, Acebo, & Carskadon, 2005). Hence, TranS-C includes interventions for increasing the homeostatic drive to sleep. When we talk about this second process with clients, it is often helpful to refer to the homeostatic process as the "hunger," "drive," or "appetite" for sleep. Homeostatic sleep drive can also be likened to a rubber band: the longer you stretch it, the more powerfully it snaps back.

In addition to incorporating the two-process model of sleep regulation, TranS-C also incorporates three empirically supported treatments to optimize sleep as well as the functioning of, and interaction between, the circadian and homeostatic processes.

Cognitive-Behavioral Therapy for Insomnia

CBT-I is a multicomponent treatment that typically comprises and incorporates one or more of the following interventions: stimulus control, sleep restriction, sleep education, relaxation therapy, and cognitive restructuring for unhelpful beliefs about sleep (Morin & Espie, 2003; Perlis, Smith, Jungquist, & Posner, 2005). Robust evidence supporting the efficacy of CBT-I comes from multiple meta-analyses (Irwin, Cole, & Nicassio, 2006; Morin, Culbert, & Schwartz,

1994; Murtagh & Greenwood, 1995; Smith et al., 2002) and systematic reviews of CBT-I in adults (Morin et al., 2006; Qaseem, Kansagara, Forciea, Cooke, & Denberg, 2016). As we have reviewed elsewhere (Harvey, 2016), the evidence for CBT-I among adolescents is limited but very promising (Bootzin & Stevens, 2005; Cassoff, Knäuper, Michaelsen, & Gruber, 2013; de Bruin, Oort, Bögels, & Meijer, 2014; Gradisar, Dohnt, et al., 2011; Paine & Gradisar, 2011; Schlarb, Liddle, & Hautzinger, 2010). This strong evidence base justified including CBT-I in TranS-C. In particular, TranS-C draws on the CBT-I components that increase homeostatic pressure to sleep and that reinforce entrainment by regular wake-up times (stimulus control and sleep restriction) and reduced arousal (cognitive therapy). In other words, TranS-C utilizes behavioral strategies to improve sleep that draw upon the two-process model of sleep regulation.

Behavioral Treatment of Circadian Rhythm Sleep–Wake Disorder, Delayed Sleep Phase Type

An evening circadian tendency refers to people who follow a delayed sleep schedule ("night owls"); they increase activity later in the day, and both go to sleep and wake up later. This broader spectrum of *eveningness* is very common, and its extreme end is represented by circadian rhythm sleep–wake disorder, delayed sleep phase type (DSPT; Lovato, Gradisar, Short, Dohnt, & Micic, 2013). DSPT is defined by sleep complaints that result from misalignment between the sleep–wake rhythm of the client and the sleep–wake schedule required by the environment. The sleep complaints of DSPT may include not being able to fall asleep until the early hours in the morning, sleeping into the next day, and being unable to sleep at "socially normal" times (American Psychiatric Association, 2013).

To address the extreme end of delayed sleep as well as the broader spectrum, TranS-C draws on research on DSPT (Gradisar, Dohnt, et al., 2011; Gradisar, Smits, & Bjorvatn, 2014; Okawa, Uchiyama, Ozaki, Shibui, & Ichikawa, 1998; Regestein & Monk, 1995), including practice parameters (Sack et al., 2007) that review positive evidence for timed light exposure (with a light box), reduced light in the evening, and planned, regular sleep schedules (chronotherapy) in adults. TranS-C includes the latter two interventions, with two important adaptations. First, many people are not motivated to use a light box, and purchasing a light box involves some additional expense. Hence, TranS-C aims to help clients develop lifelong habits of natural morning light exposure and evening dim light through electronic curfews. Second, traditional phase-delay chronotherapy involves progressively delaying bedtimes and wake times until the desired alignment is reached. Unfortunately, this type of treatment is highly disruptive to family and work schedules. Therefore, in TranS-C we often adopt a protocol that involves setting bedtimes earlier by 20–30 minutes per week. This slower approach is based on our clinical experience and the realization that our circadian system adapts more slowly to earlier bedtimes than to later ones. We have found this schedule to be achievable and a source of accomplishment and mastery for the client, which further increases the motivation for change. However, more research is needed to establish the ideal sleep modification for various groups of clients that balances circadian and motivational processes.

Interpersonal and Social Rhythm Therapy

Interpersonal and social rhythm therapy (IPSRT) is a treatment approach derived from the "social zeitgeber" theory of depression. This theory hypothesizes that life stresses disrupt our daily and social rhythms, which can lead to pathological entrainment of our circadian system. Given that moods are regulated in part by circadian processes, pathological entrainment can, in vulnerable individuals, lead to depression or other mood episodes (Ehlers, Frank, & Kupfer, 1988). IPSRT includes strategies that are designed to develop and maintain stability in social rhythms, and that draw from both human and animal research showing that the sleep and circadian systems are surprisingly sensitive to nonphotic cues, including physical activity, feeding times, and social interaction. IPSRT emphasizes stabilizing these daily rhythms to help stabilize the sleep–wake schedule. A robust evidence base for stabilizing circadian rhythms with IPSRT in bipolar disorder and depression has developed (Frank et al., 2005; Hlastala, Kotler, McClellan, & McCauley, 2010; Miklowitz et al., 2007).

Many people have irregular social and personal schedules and irregular sleep–wake cycles. In particular, adolescents and young adults wake early on weekdays for school, college, or work and then sleep in on weekends (Hysing, Pallesen, Stormark, Lundervold, & Sivertsen, 2013). Many adults, particularly those who are not working, develop habits of irregular bedtimes and wake times. Irregular sleep schedules can result in a chronically "jet-lagged" or poorly entrained state to which the human circadian system cannot adjust. Accordingly, TranS-C includes aspects of IPSRT designed to stabilize sleep and wake rhythms, as well as other social rhythms (e.g., mealtimes, socializing, exercising, etc.), drawing from the treatment manual developed by Ellen Frank (2005).

TranS-C also borrows from evidence-based approaches to treating nightmares and sleep apnea and improving motivation to change. Specifically, the module for nightmares employs imagery rehearsal therapy and is based on research by Barry Krakow, Anne Germain, and their colleagues (Germain, Shear, Hall, & Buysse, 2007; Krakow et al., 2001). The module for promoting adherence to treatments for sleep apnea is derived from evidence-based approaches (Aloia et al., 2007; Bartlett, 2011a, 2011b; Means & Edinger, 2011).

Motivational interviewing (MI) tools are used throughout (Miller & Rollnick, 2013).

A Modular Treatment

We adopted a modularized approach for TranS-C for several reasons, the most important of which is that not all clients experience all types of sleep problems. We designed a modular format consisting of core and optional modules that allow the treatment sessions to be focused on the specific sleep problem experienced by each client. The modular format proved to be more time efficient and focused on each individual client's presenting problem. We were influenced in part by the work of John Weisz, Bruce Chorpita, and their colleagues in a different field, who tested the modular approach to therapy for children with anxiety, depression, or conduct problems (MATCH; e.g., Weisz et al., 2012). They randomly assigned community clinicians to deliver usual care, standard manualized disorder-focused treatment (i.e., CBT for depression, CBT for anxiety, and behavioral parent training for conduct problems) or a modular treatment that integrated the procedures from the three separate standard treatments. MATCH was associated with the best outcomes in the form of steeper trajectories of improvement and more sustained improvement relative to both usual care and to standard manualized disorder-focused treatment (Park et al., 2016; Weisz et al., 2012). Two other findings from this research program are striking. First, therapist attitudes to evidence-based treatment were more positive following the training in the modular protocol relative to the standard protocol (Borntrager, Chorpita, Higa-McMillan, & Weisz, 2009). Second, after treating cases with the modular protocol, standard protocol, and usual care, 77 therapists reported that they were more satisfied with the modular treatment, relative to the standard treatment and usual care (Chorpita et al., 2015). In summary, we felt there were excellent reasons to adopt a modular approach for TranS-C, particularly given that our goal was to develop an approach that maximizes transportability and usefulness to front-line providers.

An Overview of TranS-C

As summarized in Box 1.2, and described in the sections that follow, TranS-C consists of three sets of modules: four cross-cutting modules, four core modules, and seven optional modules. The sessions last 50 minutes and 4 to 10 sessions are typically sufficient depending on the complexity of the presentation and the number of modules to be delivered.

BOX 1.2. TranS-C Modules

Cross-cutting modules (introduced in Sessions 1–3 and featured in all sessions thereafter)				Module topics in the TranS-C intervention	Treatment module
Case Formulation	Education	Behavior Change and Motivation	Goal Setting	Establishing regular sleep–wake times	Core Module 1, Part A
				Learning a wind-down routine	Core Module 1, Part B
				Learning a wake-up routine	Core Module 1, Part C
				Improving daytime functioning	Core Module 2
				Correcting unhelpful sleep-related beliefs	Core Module 3
				Improving sleep efficiency	Optional Module 1
				Reducing time in bed	Optional Module 2
				Dealing with delayed or advanced phase	Optional Module 3
				Reducing sleep-related worry and vigilance	Optional Module 4
				Promoting compliance with the CPAP machine/exposure therapy for claustrophobic reactions	Optional Module 5
				Negotiating sleep in a complicated environment	Optional Module 6
				Reducing nightmares	Optional Module 7
				Maintenance of behavior change	Core Module 4

Cross-Cutting Modules

TranS-C includes four cross-cutting modules: Case Formulation, Sleep and Circadian Education, Behavior Change and Motivation, and Goal Setting. These are *typically* introduced in Sessions 1–3. Thereafter they become *rolling interventions* woven into every subsequent session, as described in the next sections.

Cross-Cutting Module 1: Case Formulation

Judith Beck (2011) reminds us of the value of an "ever evolving formulation," which unfolds throughout all sessions. The initial case formulation in TranS-C is based on at least a week of completed sleep diaries along with the measures described in Chapter 2 and the functional analysis described in Chapter 3. In each subsequent session, a new week's sleep diary is collected and more information about the client's sleep and circadian functioning becomes apparent as the various interventions are implemented. This new information can change or improve the accuracy of the formulation and treatment goals discussed in early treatment sessions.

Cross-Cutting Module 2: Sleep and Circadian Education

Sleep and circadian education lays the scientific foundation for the interventions that comprise TranS-C. If a client understands the science behind a recommendation, he or she is much more likely to try it. For example, many people enjoy using technology before bedtime. One client with a severe mental illness, who lives in a board and care home, described her TV as "my only friend." She slept with the TV on all night. It was positioned next to her bed, near her pillow. However, this client was willing to try turning the TV off when she learned that bright light and intermittent noise interfere with the biology of sleep. Sleep and circadian education becomes a "rolling intervention" in two ways: (1) most of the core and optional modules include an education component that provides an opportunity to review and extend the information covered in this early phase of treatment, and (2) it is important to provide regular reminders of the sleep and circadian education as they help the client recall the rationale for each intervention. For example, a client may note that, surprisingly, she slept better after needing to get up early for an appointment that morning. This could be pointed out to her as an example of increased homeostatic sleep drive from waking earlier, contributing to better sleep the following night.

Cross-Cutting Module 3: Behavior Change and Motivation

Facilitating the client's adoption of healthy sleep habits is difficult. Behavior change is challenging for everyone, not just for those who have sleep problems. For example, if you made a New Year's resolution, do you remember what the resolution is? Have you achieved it? Most New Year's resolutions are forgotten. MI and related behavior change strategies should be reflexively folded into every session, particularly when homework for the coming week is being planned.

Cross-Cutting Module 4: Goal Setting

Client sleep goals provide a focus for treatment and for monitoring progress. Goals are set for both the night and the day. The daytime goals are important given that daytime impairment is an essential feature of sleep problems (American Academy of Sleep Medicine, 2005; American Psychiatric Association, 2013; Edinger, Bonnet, et al., 2004). Therapy goals are set in the early sessions of TranS-C, but they may need to be reevaluated and readjusted periodically as the intervention unfolds.

Core Modules

TranS-C also includes four core modules that apply to the vast majority of clients.

Core Module 1: Establishing Regular Sleep–Wake Times

Regularity is a core dimension of the sleep health framework, (Buysse, 2014). To establish regularity, the first part of this module is based on IPSRT (Frank et al., 2005; Frank, Swartz, & Kupfer, 2000) and stimulus control (Bootzin, 1972) principles. The second and third parts of this module include working with the client to plan a personalized wind-down routine before bedtime and a wake-up routine in the morning. These latter two modules support the process of establishing regular sleep–wake times.

Core Module 2: Improving Daytime Functioning

This module teaches strategies to improve daytime functioning with a focus on skills for coping with a night of poor sleep. Nighttime and daytime impairment can be at least partly functionally independent (Lichstein, Durrence, Riedel, &

Bayen, 2001; Neitzert Semler & Harvey, 2005). Thus, TranS-C includes separate strategies to help clients improve their nighttime sleep and their daytime functioning.

Core Module 3: Correcting Unhelpful Sleep-Related Beliefs

Holding unhelpful beliefs about sleep is common. This module uses education, guided discovery, and individualized experiments to address unhelpful beliefs about sleep. Several studies show that a reduction in unhelpful beliefs about sleep after treatment for insomnia is associated with persistent, enduring improvements in sleep (Edinger, Wohlgemuth, Radtke, Marsh, & Quillian, 2001; Morin, Blais, & Savard, 2002).

Core Module 4: Maintenance of Behavior Change

This module is designed to consolidate gains and ensure for setbacks using an individualized summary of learning and achievements. Therapist and client start preparing for this module by reviewing and charting progress, checking on goal attainment, identifying specific problem areas that need more attention, and summarizing the learning that has taken place over the course of treatment.

Optional Modules

There are seven optional modules that are used, depending on the needs of each client, and we provide guidance on deciding when to use each of them. While the order of the treatment components for each of the modules is broadly suggestive of the order of completion, it is important to be sensitive to the differences between clients as to which processes are maintaining their distress and to address those processes at an earlier stage of treatment. Of course, the therapist should not move from one treatment component to another until the client is ready. This approach recognizes that each client will move through the different stages of treatment at a different pace.

Optional Module 1: Improving Sleep Efficiency

Sleep efficiency is one of the six dimensions of healthy sleep. Too much time in bed spent not sleeping indicates sleep inefficiency. The extensive insomnia literature shows that two components of CBT-I are particularly effective for improving sleep efficiency: stimulus control and sleep restriction (Morin et al., 2006).

Optional Module 2: Reducing Time in Bed

Spending too much time in bed is a problem. It can impair one's ability to live life fully and makes it difficult to fully engage with work, family, and friends. It is also associated with more emotional disturbance, unhappiness, and interpersonal problems, more substance abuse, excessive daytime sleepiness, and impairment in daily activities and level of productivity (Kaplan, Gruber, Eidelman, Talbot, & Harvey, 2011). It is possible that too much time in bed will have an adverse impact on health because the human body has evolved to spend two-thirds of each day awake and active. As mentioned earlier, sleep duration and sleep efficiency are two of the dimensions of the sleep health framework (Buysse, 2014). Interventions include education on sleep inertia, assessing and problem-solving why the client spends so much time in bed, setting daytime goals, and developing strategies for managing low energy and fatigue.

Optional Module 3: Dealing with Delayed or Advanced Phase

This module is relevant if sleep is later or earlier than is preferred by the client. TranS-C includes shifting the timing of light and other zeitgebers earlier or later depending on the phase; for example, dim light, an electronic curfew, and progressively moving to an earlier bedtime for the delayed phase or a later bedtime for the advanced phase.

Optional Module 4: Reducing Sleep-Related Worry and Vigilance

People with sleep problems often worry while trying to get to sleep at the beginning of the night, after waking in the middle of the night, and on waking too early in the morning. Anxiety is antithetical to sleep (Espie, 2002), and because excessive worry and rumination fuel anxiety and arousal, it is important to teach these clients skills to manage their unwanted thoughts. A range of skills are taught, including how to identify and evaluate negative thoughts, practicing gratitude and savoring, setting a worry time, problem solving, journaling, and using pleasant imagery.

Optional Module 5: Promoting Compliance with the Continuous Positive Airway Pressure Machine/Exposure Therapy for Claustrophobic Reactions

While TranS-C does not directly treat sleep apnea, this module helps clients with sleep apnea to adjust to using a continuous positive airway pressure (CPAP) machine when prescribed by a sleep specialist. Education and motivational strategies are used to increase CPAP machine use at night. Graded exposure is used with clients who have a claustrophobic reaction to the machine.

Optional Module 6: Negotiating Sleep in a Complicated Environment

Many environmental factors may interfere with the ability to sleep. This solution-focused module works toward minimizing the impact of these issues. The module assumes that clients have resources and strengths to resolve complaints. The emphasis is on acknowledging distress, focusing the conversation on success, and discussing solutions rather than problems—in other words, on what is possible and changeable, rather than on what is impossible and intractable (De Shazer & Dolan, 2012; Lloyd, 2008). The module draws on the evidence-based problem-solving module from Cognitive Behavioral Social Skills Training (CBSST; Granholm, Holden, Link, McQuaid, & Jeste, 2013), which involves teaching the client the *SCALE* acronym: **S**pecify the problem, **C**onsider all possible solutions, **A**ssess the best solution, **L**ay out a plan, and **E**xecute and **E**valuate the outcome as an approach to solving problems. Communication skills are taught through role playing.

Optional Module 7: Reducing Nightmares

Nightmares are disturbing because the content of the dream or the emotions in the dream are unpleasant, and these features persist after the sleeper awakens. Seventy-five to 90% of people who experience stressful life events report nightmares; most people have experienced a nightmare at least once in their life. This module is based on research by Barry Krakow, Anne Germain, and their colleagues (Germain et al., 2007; Krakow et al., 2001). The evidence base for treating nightmares with imagery rehearsal therapy is strong. It results in a significant reduction in the number of nightmares per week and in improved sleep. Interestingly, imagery rehearsal therapy is also associated with a decrease in PTSD symptoms (Casement & Swanson, 2012).

Who Is Qualified to Conduct TranS-C?

The ideal providers of TranS-C are individuals who have training and experience conducting CBT and MI and who have a working knowledge of the biology of sleep. Having said that, we have successfully trained people who have minimal knowledge of CBT and sleep to become outstanding TranS-C providers after having more intensive training and supervision that focuses on giving them extensive feedback on recorded sessions.

Who Is an Appropriate Client for TranS-C?

With developmental adaptations, as described throughout this book, we have been delivering TranS-C to treat sleep disturbance in youth 10 years or older through to older adults. In addition, we have been using TranS-C to treat sleep problems for both mental and physical illnesses. Clearly, the approach takes seriously the task of solving the "too many empirically supported treatments problem" (Weisz et al., 2014, p. 68).

More specifically, as part of a study funded by the National Institute of Child Health and Human Development (NICHD), we have been delivering this approach to 10- to 18-year-olds with a broad range of sleep problems, particularly teens who are night owls. Among youth, insomnia is a common sleep problem (Buysse et al., 2008; Gradisar, Gardner, et al., 2011). However, insomnia often overlaps with features of hypersomnia, difficulty getting up in the morning, sleepiness during the day, inadequate opportunity to sleep, irregular sleep–wake schedules, worry and rumination about social concerns (e.g., dating, getting into college) and worry and rumination about not sleeping. Accordingly, we have included adaptations to address this broad range of sleep disturbances effectively and efficiently.

In adults, as part of a study funded by the National Institute of Mental Health (NIMH), we have also delivered TranS-C to clients with a severe mental illness in a community mental health setting. The clients have a broad range of diagnoses, particularly schizophrenia, bipolar disorder, posttraumatic stress disorder (PTSD), and depression as well as comorbid medical problems. In this study, clients continue to take their usual medications. Interestingly, in an earlier study modifying CBT-I for those with bipolar disorder (BP) (Harvey et al., 2015), more clients in the CBTI-BP group than clients in the psychoeducation group were able to discontinue at least one sleep medication at some point during the treatment phase (66.7% vs. 29.4%; $p = 0.04$). Also, Buysse and colleagues (2011) conducted a large randomized controlled trial of a brief behavioral treatment for older adults with chronic insomnia; clients on medications were included and there was no difference in outcomes among clients taking or not taking sleep medications. Considering these studies together, we are confident that TranS-C can be delivered concurrently with usual medications.

Flexibility, Adaptation, and Balance

Box 1.2 broadly represents the order in which modules are typically completed. However, as we pointed out earlier, it is important to be aware of which processes maintain a client's distress and to address those processes at an earlier treatment stage, keeping in mind that clients make progress at different rates. Some clients quickly grasp the sleep and circadian education module that forms the rationale for TranS-C. However, other clients do better when the therapist divides up this module across multiple sessions and flexibly adapts the material to optimally match the client's concerns and interests. The selection and sequencing of modules typically become apparent during the case formulation (Cross-Cutting Module 1, described in Chapter 3). For example, one client began the first session by telling the therapist, "I am a hopeless case. I have tried every treatment for my sleep problem. Nothing works. I am sorry but I am wasting your time." In this case, moving the thinking traps intervention within Optional Module 4 to Session 2 effectively encouraged the client to give TranS-C a try. Another client was worried about trying the recommended sleep adjustments. She said, "I will fail for sure. Then I will disappoint you." In this case, we moved the negative automatic thoughts portion of Optional Module 4 to Session 2. Evaluating the thoughts "I will fail for sure. Then I will disappoint you" with the Evaluating Negative Automatic Thoughts form (Appendix 15) was helpful for reducing the fear of failure.

When selecting which parts of TranS-C to emphasize, we advise providing a balanced perspective and using the material in this book flexibly, adapting it as needed for each client. For example, clients who have been encouraged (or forced!) to come to treatment by a parent/guardian, doctor, or a case manager can sometimes be relatively happy with their (poor) sleep and are unmotivated to change. For these clients, we prioritize spending time explaining the health consequences of poor sleep. Also, as the therapist gets to know each client, other motivations for change typically become apparent. For example, an adolescent client might care about getting good grades to get into college. In this case we would discuss in some detail the link between academic performance and sleep, and remind the teen of the link throughout the sessions. For clients who are very anxious about their sleep, we would not emphasize the health consequences of poor sleep, given that this will likely exacerbate anxiety and therefore the sleep problem. Instead, we would prioritize the modules that are most helpful for reducing anxiety (e.g., Core Module 3, Optional Module 4). Another common example are clients who are perfectionists. These clients sometimes need to devote *less effort* to sleeping, as described in Core Module 3, and prescribing rigid rules only adds to the long list of rigid rules they are already living by. Interestingly, Buysse et al. (2010) showed that people diagnosed with insomnia (who are often anxious too) have irregular wake times, but they are actually a bit more regular in terms of their bedtimes compared to people without a sleep problem. For people who present with this pattern, consider suggesting more flexible sleep–wake times. In other words, instead of recommending a specific time to go to bed and wake up, consider the recommendation "Go to bed no *earlier* than _____, and get out of bed no *later* than _____."

Session Structure

Box 1.3 lists the basic session structure for TranS-C, and its main parts are briefly described next.

Set the Agenda

Following an introduction of the general CBT principles, every session begins by setting an agenda. Say what you would like to do in the session, check whether your agenda is acceptable to the client, and ask the client if anything needs to be added to the agenda. Be careful that the agenda set at the beginning of the session doesn't get long and boring. Try to add excitement and inspiration to your tone of voice and to the content of the agenda—for example: "Sleep is *so* interesting. I am very excited to share some information on the science behind why and how we sleep."

Ask the Client for Feedback on the Previous Session

Typically the next agenda item is to ask for feedback on the previous session and provide memory support for the content of last session. For example, "It's been about a week since we met. Did we do anything or did I say anything

---

BOX 1.3. Basic Session Structure

- Set the session agenda.
- Review the previous session with the client.
- Review and comment on the daily sleep diary.
  - How regular or irregular are the bedtimes and wake times across the 7 days?
  - Any long sleep onset latencies? How long?
  - Any long awakenings after sleep onset? How long?
  - Any snoozing in the morning after wake time?
  - How many awakenings during the night? For how long?
  - Any naps?
- Review the goals and homework assigned in the previous session.
- Work on the client's main problems.
- Set goals and give homework for the next week.
- Ask the client to summarize the session.
- Ask for feedback on the session.

that was particularly helpful or unhelpful?"; "Thinking back to our last session, what stood out to you the most?" It doesn't matter if the client can't remember anything; the therapist should then chime in with the two to three points that are most helpful to remember. This practice promotes encoding of the main contents of treatment (Harvey et al., 2014).

Review and Comment on the Daily Sleep Diary

The client should bring the completed sleep diary to every session. It is an important source of information about current sleep habits and the effect of suggested interventions. Reviewing the diary may directly lead into new treatment recommendations.

Review Goals and Homework Assigned in the Previous Session

Did your client complete the homework or achieve the goal? What did he or she learn? If not, why not?

Work on the Client's Main Problems

Incorporate frequent summaries using simple language. Use a white board or paper tablet when relevant. Use in-session and between-session behavioral experiments. The client or therapist can write a brief summary of the session's main points for the client to take home.

Set Goals and Homework for the Next Week

We strongly recommend having a written copy of any assignments for clients to take home to help them remember. Make a clear rationale for each item on the homework list and how the assignment's activity relates to the client's goals for therapy. Begin the assigned activity in session by practicing the skills, anticipating the difficulties, and asking the client, "What things might prevent you from doing this?" Reinforce the value of the home project by asking, "Any thoughts about how you might use this information you gather from this?"; "Can you think of anything that will prevent you from doing it?"; "How could you answer that thought at the time?"; "What could we plan now that might overcome that problem?"

Ask the Client to Summarize the Session

Ask the client what are the main points or what she or he has learned—for example: "Was there anything that stood out that you want to be sure to remember?" Help the client by filling in the gaps.

Ask for Feedback on the Session

Check whether there was anything in the session that was unsatisfactory or unhelpful. Ask for feedback about how it went—for example: "Did we do anything or did I say anything that was particularly helpful or unhelpful?"

Key Interventions Used in TranS-C

Education about Sleep

In addition to the support provided in Chapter 3, we provide several categories of accompanying materials, or handouts, that provide the client with education about sleep. These handouts are contained in Appendices 4, 5, and 8. Working through these handouts collaboratively with the client can generate talking points and prompts to help you cover several of the main topics. Also a list of helpful videos available on the Internet (Appendix 2) and various other forms of media (Appendix 1) are particularly helpful for catching the client's attention and breaking up more didactic portions of the session.

Behavioral Experiments

Bennett-Levy et al. (2004) define behavioral experiments as

> planned experiential activities, based on experimentation or observation, which are undertaken by clients in or between . . . therapy sessions. Their design is derived directly from a . . . formulation of the problem, and their primary purpose is to obtain new information which . . . [includes] . . . contributing to the development and verification of the . . . formulation. (p. 8)

Behavioral experiments encourage clients to make judgments in their lives based on data they collect, as scientists do, rather than based solely on their subjective feelings.

We suggest setting up experiments during the course of TranS-C and provide examples of such experiments in subsequent chapters. Very often, conducting one simple behavioral experiment brings about a profound disconfirmation of unhelpful beliefs or stunning demonstrations that certain behaviors or thoughts are important contributors to the sleep problem. Behavioral experiments are much more powerful for facilitating change than verbal discussions of the same topic (Harvey, Clark, Ehlers, & Rapee, 2000; Tang & Harvey, 2004). They offer deep experiential learning that new thoughts, beliefs, and behaviors can reduce anxiety and improve sleep. Indeed, in TranS-C we consider each client to be a budding sleep scientist. This approach also encourages a curiosity and sense of adventure that often generates a willingness to try a new behavior "just once." Quite often, this experiment is enough to kick-start the building blocks of a new, healthier habit.

There are endless possibilities for behavioral experiments for sleep problems. As discussed in subsequent chapters, some experiments are conducted *within a session* and others are given as homework to be conducted *between sessions.* The latter can be facilitated with text or email support from the therapist (e.g., the client might text the therapist the result of the experiment soon after completing it). Some experiments involve observation (e.g., the survey experiment described in Core Module 3), whereas other experiments involve an experimental manipulation (e.g., the energy experiment described in Core Module 2). Also, some experiments are thought experiments, while other experiments involve a change in behavior.

As specified by Bennett-Levy et al. (2004), there are six steps to completing a behavioral experiment: (1) precisely identify the belief, thought, or process; (2) brainstorm ideas for an experiment to test the thought or belief (very specific); (3) make predictions about the outcome and devise a method to record the outcome; (4) anticipate problems and brainstorm solutions; (5) conduct the experiment; and (6) review the experiment and draw conclusions. Additional tips for behavioral experiments are presented in Box 1.4.

CBT Skills

The therapist skill of guided discovery is crucial in TranS-C. Therapist questions can encourage the client to use their current knowledge and experience to piece together and discover things or piece together evidence in a new way. The stance of the therapist is collaborative and curious, using questioning to help the client to look at situations in various ways and to help the client to draw his or her own conclusions. We encourage readers who are unfamiliar with these skills to refer to CBT resources where these skills are taught in detail (J. S. Beck, 2011; Greenberger & Padesky, 2016; Wells, 1997).

Stimulus Control and Sleep Restriction

These interventions are used when the client has become conditioned to associate the bed or bedroom with being awake and anxious about not sleeping. Stimulus control and sleep restriction are designed to break the bed–not sleeping link and restore the bed–sleep link. In stimulus control, developed by Richard Bootzin and colleagues (Bootzin, Epstein, & Wood, 1991), the client is to go to bed only when sleepy, use the bed only for sleep and sex, and get out of bed if he or she is not falling asleep. The basic idea behind sleep restriction, developed by Arthur Spielman and colleagues (Spielman, Saskin, & Thorpy,

BOX 1.4. Tips for Behavioral Experiments

When developing a behavioral experiment:

- Conduct a *thorough assessment* of the domain you are targeting. For example, don't target caffeine if you don't know your client's pattern of caffeine use.

- Make the experiment *consistent with a goal* you and your client have agreed to work on together. For example, don't target caffeine if your client is not on board with reducing caffeine use.

- *Make the experiment brief or once only.* Many clients are more likely to give a new sleep pattern a try if it is set up as an experiment for just *one day* or *one weekend*. Often one experience of the new sleep pattern is enough to convince the client to consider using the new strategy habitually.

- *Consider offering between-session support.* We often offer between-session support for experiments. For example, in working on a wind-down routine, you could text the client at the "switch time" (the time the person has decided that he or she would like to switch into his or her wind-down routine) for a few nights in the hope that this approach helps to build an action tendency for the person to make the switch on his or her own. Future research is needed to determine how many nights are needed to create an "action tendency."

- *Do not focus on unrealistic outcomes.* Clients may not immediately feel better when they change their sleep patterns for the following reasons:
  - Some clients respond to sleep deprivation with hypomania, so they may feel better in certain ways when they are not getting enough sleep.
  - Clients' feelings (e.g., tiredness) may have become the norm. It might take time for this habit to change.
  - Clients may confuse feelings of tiredness with feelings of boredom.
  - If clients have been habitually sleep deprived or have habitually had irregular sleep and wake times, it can take 1–3 weeks to realign their biological clocks before they notice feeling better. Thus, if you make "feeling more alert" the outcome of a behavioral experiment, consider explaining to the client why this change may not be observed right away.

1987), is that time in bed should be limited to maximize the sleep drive, so that the association between the bed and sleeping is strengthened. It begins by reducing the time spent in bed. More detailed instructions can be found in Optional Module 1.

Additional Interventions

Other interventions include exposure for clients who have phobic reactions to using the CPAP machine (Optional Module 5), role playing for teaching communication skills to help clients negotiate sleep in a complicated environment (Optional Module 6), and imagery rehearsal therapy for reducing nightmares (Optional Module 7).

Working with Parents and Caregivers of Adolescent Clients

The increasing independence of adolescents means that when delivering TranS-C to youth we are principally youth focused. Nonetheless, parents and caregivers can often help to promote an acceptance and reinforcement of treatment-mediated changes and keep their child enrolled in treatment. In those families with unhealthy dynamics, maintaining contact with the parents can help the clinician to circumvent them from subtly undermining sleep changes. Our focus is to orient parents toward positively reinforcing their teen for establishing a regularized sleep–wake cycle and assisting their teen *when invited.* When developmentally appropriate, we typically invite parents to join the final 5–10 minutes at the end of each session. In this time, the teen (assisted by the therapist) gives a summary of the session and the plan for the coming week and might ask for specific forms of help from their caregiver. However, we have learned to go with teens' wishes when they do not want to bring their parents or caregivers into the session. Particularly for older youth, there can be much conflict at home around sleep. It is better to not bring these issues into the therapy room. Instead, place phone calls to the parent(s) between sessions.

We have also found it very helpful to ask about the schedule of the parents, siblings, and other people who live in the house, as described in the following examples.

> A client's father worked an evening shift and then enjoyed special time with his daughter in the later evening. Knowing the father's schedule was important for negotiating with the father and daughter to find an earlier bedtime. We moved the special father–daughter time to Saturday morning brunch as an incentive to help the daughter get up in the morning, while also helping her to get to sleep earlier on weeknights.

We worked out a morning schedule with a client that upset the client's mother because it meant that she would be 30 minutes late for work. We should have checked with the client's mother about her schedule first.

When talking to parents and caregivers, we suggest trying to:

- Emphasize the importance of their teen's regular attendance at sessions.
- Emphasize the importance of their teen's completion of the sleep diary.
- Elicit motivational statements.
- Help develop plans for overcoming barriers to treatment that may arise.
- Clarify their role.
- Share sleep-related resources they may find interesting or helpful.

See the handout we give parents on their role in their teen's sleep treatment in Appendix 12.

No One Sleeps Perfectly All the Time

The ongoing emphasis throughout TranS-C is that everyone has a bad night of sleep sometimes, particularly when stressed, and this is normal. One of the aims is to equip clients with tools and methods to help them continue to improve their sleep and cope with an occasional night of poor sleep once therapy is over. An explanation of normal sleep can be helpful, noting that everyone usually wakes up at night, and everyone has some variability in their sleep from night to night. The survey experiment described in Core Module 3 can help a client to grasp the reality of a normal night of sleep.

Plan of this Book

This chapter has introduced TranS-C, outlined the theoretical and clinical principles that are core to TranS-C, and presented an overview of its modules and structure. The next chapter focuses on the initial assessment of clients who present with a sleep problem. The assessment helps to determine which clients are appropriate for TranS-C and instructs therapists on how to deliver TranS-C. Chapters 3, 4, and 5 describe the cross-cutting modules, core modules, and optional modules that comprise TranS-C, respectively. An epilogue is devoted to summarizing the approach and outlining future directions.

CHAPTER 2

Sleep Assessment

The goal of this chapter is to provide an overview of the assessment of a broad range of sleep problems. First, we begin by offering some guidance on how to conduct a sleep history clinical interview. Second, we describe the methods we suggest using to obtain a baseline assessment and to measure progress across TranS-C. In selecting the measures, we prioritized brief measures to reduce the burden on clients, and we prioritized instruments with strong psychometric properties. Third, we include brief descriptions of the most common sleep disorders, noting those that are covered by TranS-C and those that should trigger a referral to a sleep specialist. Finally, we describe several additional assessments of sleep that are important to know about when working with clients who have sleep and circadian problems.

A current unmet need in the field is the availability of developmentally adapted sleep and circadian measures for youth. Throughout this chapter, we note the domains for which we are aware of a youth-specific measure. If measures that have been developed and validated for adults are used to assess youth, care should be taken to interpret the results in a way that respects the recommendation that most youth obtain 8½–9½ hours per night. The current recommendation for adults is 7–8 hours of sleep per night. Older adults should aim for around 7 hours of sleep per night.

Sleep History Clinical Interview

Predominant Complaint

The clinical interview (Harvey & Spielman, 2011) starts by determining which of the following complaints is predominant for the client:

- Not enough sleep
- Trouble falling asleep
- Difficulty staying asleep
- Early morning awakening
- Light or nonrefreshing sleep
- Unable to sleep without sleeping pills
- Sleeping too much
- Sleeping at inconvenient times of the day
- Sleep that is unpredictable

We also assess for sleep disorders that are associated with too little sleep (i.e., insomnia), too much sleep, sleep at unusual times (i.e., circadian rhythm disorders), and sleep with unusual experiences (i.e., parasomnias, movements disorders, and sleep apnea) (American Academy of Sleep Medicine, 2014; American Psychiatric Association, 2013).

Frequency, Variability, Sleep Habits

Next, we ask the client more specific questions about the frequency of the problem and the night-to-night variability (Spielman & Anderson, 1999). Other topics to systematically work through with clients are the sleep habits they have developed, including:

- The time the client gets into bed. (Many clients go to bed very early in an attempt to maximize the amount of sleep they obtain.)
- The activities engaged in once in bed.
- The time of lights out (including how the decision to turn the lights out is made).
- Sleep onset latency (the difference between the time of lights out and the time of falling asleep).
- Awakenings (the number, timing, and duration; the client's experience of awakenings, particularly any distress they cause and how the client copes).
- Wake-up time (could be determined by environmental disturbances and can be variable or unvarying; the latter is suggestive of a circadian component to the insomnia).
- Out-of-bed time. (Does the client linger in bed and occasionally fall back to sleep? If so, this is suggestive of poor sleep hygiene.)
- Total sleep time (TST) (Does it vary on the weekdays vs. the weekends?).

In addition, assessing sleep and daytime functioning before the onset of the sleep problem can provide helpful information.

Daytime Functioning

Daytime impairment is an essential feature of sleep disorders (American Academy of Sleep Medicine, 2005; American Psychiatric Association, 2013; Edinger, Bonnet, et al., 2004). As such, we include an assessment of the impact of the sleep problem on daytime functioning covering work, social life, family life, and recreational activities.

Psychiatric History

We also recommend that comorbid psychiatric disorders be assessed with the Structured Clinical Interview for DSM Disorders (SCID) or a psychiatric history, along with questionnaire measures of mood, such as the Inventory of Depressive Symptomatology (IDS) or the Beck Depression Inventory II (BDI-II) and the State–Trait Anxiety Inventory for Adults (STAI-AD). For youth, we use the Children's Depression Rating Scale (CDRS) and the Multidimensional Anxiety Scale for Children (MASC; or similar). Mood questionnaires are singled out, since mood disorders are the most common comorbid conditions.

Medical History and Sleep Medications

Pain, discomfort, and treatment side effects associated with medical disorders are often problematic for having a healthy sleep; therefore an assessment of a client's medical history, current health, and medication use is essential. For medications we obtain information about the type, amount, time of administration, frequency of use, side effects, withdrawal effects on discontinuation, and degree of tolerance. When taking a history of sleep medication use, be sure to ask how and when the client decides to take the medication. If he or she starts the night by trying to fall asleep without a sleeping pill and then lies in bed worrying about whether or not sleep will come and whether or not to take a pill, the client may wait several hours, then take a pill and suffer sedating effects on waking. Conversely, many clients take sleeping pills too early, when they are not even sleepy, thinking that the pill will make them so. There are several problems with this decision. It gives a lot more power to the pill than is realistic; sleeping pills don't make a wide-awake person go to sleep. Second, this practice can lead people to take sleeping pills far too early, so that the peak level of the medication occurs before a natural/reasonable sleep time. Third, it allows the medication to be taken far before the sleep drive has reached its peak, thus decoupling two potentially useful promoters of sleep onset.

Assessment of Sleep and Circadian Function

The PROMIS Sleep Disturbance (Buysse et al., 2010; Yu, Buysse, Germain, & Moul, 2012) and the PROMIS Sleep-Related Impairment scales (Buysse et al., 2010; Yu et al., 2012) are brief, comprehensive, and well-validated measures of nighttime and daytime impairment, respectively. As will become evident, sleeping in the night and functioning in the day are *both* important treatment targets in TranS-C. We use the short form (eight items) of these scales, which are scored 1 ("not at all") to 5 ("very much"). These scales are ideal for TranS-C because they are not specific to a particular diagnosis (e.g., insomnia or sleep apnea). Instead, the questions capture the broad range of sleep and circadian problems targeted by TranS-C.

The Daily Sleep Diary

The daily sleep diary is a very important tool for assessing sleep problems. Ideally, the diary is kept for at least 7–14 days prior to the beginning of TranS-C. If possible, a sleep diary can be sent to a new client at the time an appointment is scheduled, along with instructions to complete it and bring to the first session (see Appendix 13 for a blank sleep diary and instructions). Alternatively, provide the sleep diary and instructions during the first session for the client to complete before the second session and move the assessment related to the sleep diary to Session 2.

It is very important to provide each client training in how to complete the sleep diary either with written instructions or in person. If you do the training in person, go through the client's "last night," completing the diary together as an opportunity to train the client in accurately completing the diary. Be sure to distinguish the time getting into bed from the time intending to go to sleep, distinguish the last awakening from the arising time, and make sure to get the total amount of time awake after sleep onset (e.g., if a client reports three awakenings with a duration of 30 minutes, be clear on whether the 30 minutes refers to each awakening or to all three awakenings in total). Giving the client a strong rationale for the completion of the sleep diary is also very helpful; namely, the daily sleep diary is used to develop the treatment plan each week and to track treatment progress. A good rule of thumb is that completing the morning sleep diary should take no longer than 2 minutes. This is sufficient to obtain good-quality sleep diary data, while preventing an excessive focus on sleep times.

There are many different versions of sleep diaries, and they are often adapted for the needs of specific client groups (e.g., simplified for younger youth). Colleen Carney and her colleagues (2012) developed a consensus sleep diary based on expert agreement and qualitative client input (the blank sleep diary and instructions in Appendix 13 are based on this consensus sleep diary). The authors proposed that all sleep diary versions should contain "core" sleep questions to adequately address the sleep problem. Core sleep questions that should be included in the sleep diary include (1) "What time did you get into bed?"; (2) "What time did you try to go to sleep?"; (3) "How long did it take you to fall asleep?"; (4) How many times did you wake up, not counting your final awakening?"; (5) "In total, how long did these awakenings last?"; (6) "What time was your final awakening?"; (7) "What time did you get out of bed for the day?"; (8) "How would you rate the quality of your sleep (on a scale from 'poor' to 'very good')?"; and (9) "Do you have any additional comments pertaining to your sleep?" These core questions align nicely with previous recommendations as to the most important parameters to derive from the sleep diary (Buysse, Ancoli-Israel, Edinger, Lichstein, & Morin, 2006).

The client completes the sleep diary each morning at home. When the client arrives for an appointment, the therapist can quickly inspect the sleep diary to get a good sense of overall patterns, as described in the next section. However, the therapist can maximize the value of the sleep diary by completing a few additional calculations. Some of the key variables in a sleep diary are derived from these calculations. Specifically, the therapist should calculate values for time in bed (TIB), total sleep time (TST), sleep efficiency (SE), and midsleep time (MST). These values can be calculated for each day of the diary, then averaged across days or the week. Box 2.1 contains detailed instructions on how to complete these calculations. Some therapists may have resources for developing a computer program for calculating the key variables, but a regular calculator is all that's really needed.

It is often helpful to include additional questions in the sleep diary to monitor other treatment targets, such as a rating of daytime energy or nightmare occurrence. For example, questions pertaining to alcohol and caffeine use, medication use, napping, and exercise might be helpful in further analyzing the sleep problem.

One important advantage of keeping a daily sleep diary is that it reduces the effect of biases in memory and information processing. In retrospective reports that require clients to average sleep times over the past week or past month, the sleep times and amounts recorded in the sleep diary will inevitably be influenced by the most salient and the most recent nights. Recording sleep in a daily sleep diary immediately after waking can overcome this limitation.

While the completion of a paper version of the sleep diary is inexpensive and easy to use, web-based and electronic options are available (Edinger, Means, Stechuchak, & Olsen, 2004). These methods can increase efficiency and accuracy because the data are time stamped, ensuring that the diary really has been completed every morning.

BOX 2.1. Instructions to Therapists
for Calculating Key Variables from the Sleep Diary

Calculating an individual's sleep times from a sleep diary is vitally important for conducting TranS-C, but can also be a little bit tricky for three reasons: (1) time is usually measured in terms of hours and minutes, whereas calculations are much more easily done with decimals; (2) bedtimes that cross midnight cause mischief with calculations; and (3) many people do not understand the distinction between A.M. and P.M. (let alone military time!). This brief guide will help you to generate the key variables from a client's sleep diary. It may seem a little confusing at first, but with practice, it will become second nature. We would strongly advise having a calculator handy for these procedures.

To make the most use of your client's sleep diary you will need to calculate four variables:

1. *Time in bed (TIB):* The total amount of time the individual spends in bed, from the time he or she first gets into bed at night until the time she or he gets out of bed in the morning.
2. *Total sleep time (TST):* The total amount of time the individual actually spends asleep, as opposed to being awake in bed.
3. *Sleep efficiency (SE):* The ratio of TST/TIB * 100. Multiplying by 100 allows you to express sleep efficiency as a percent, specifically, the percent of time in bed actually spent sleeping.
4. *Midsleep time (MST):* The time of the middle of the sleep period, from getting into bed at night until getting out of bed in the morning.

Once you have calculated each variable for each night, you can then take an average across the week (or for however many days you have sleep diary information).

Getting Started

Sleep diary calculations become much easier if you convert hours and minutes into a total number of minutes. In order to convert hours into minutes, simply multiply the reported hours by 60:

$$\text{Minutes} = \text{Reported hours} * 60$$

So, for 6 hours:

$$\text{Minutes} = 6 \text{ hours} * 60 \text{ minutes per hour} = 360 \text{ minutes}$$

This calculation works for amounts of time (for instance, sleep latency or duration of awakenings) as well as for reported clock times. For example:

A reported sleep latency of 1:25 (1 hour, 25 minutes) =
(1 ∗ 60) minutes + 25 minutes = 60 minutes + 25 minutes = 85 minutes

A wake-up time of 6:30 A.M. = 6 hours + 30 minutes = (6 ∗ 60) + 30 =
360 + 30 = 390 minutes after midnight

One more hint to make the calculations easier: Think of clock times between midnight and noon as positive numbers. Think of clock times between noon and midnight as negative numbers. For hours between noon and midnight, simply subtract 720 from all "P.M." times in minutes. Doing this will make the calculations of TIB and MST much easier. For example:

As we saw in the above equation, a wake-up time of 6:30 A.M. =
6 hours + 30 minutes = (6 ∗ 60) + 30 = 360 + 30 = 390 minutes after midnight

A bedtime of 11:15 P.M. = [(11 hours ∗ 60 minutes per hour) + 15 minutes]
− 720 = [(660) + 15] − 720 = 675 − 720 = −45 minutes
Remember, −45 means 45 minutes before midnight

In order to convert minutes back to hours and minutes, first divide the total number of minutes by 60. Then, multiply anything after the decimal point by 60. For example:

443 minutes = 443 minutes/60 minutes per hour = 7.38 hours =
7 hours + (0.38 hours ∗ 60 minutes per hour) = 7 hours + 23 minutes = 7:23

Calculating TIB

1. Calculate bedtime in minutes.
2. Calculate time out of bed in minutes.
3. Subtract bedtime from time out of bed.

For example, suppose your client has a bedtime of 10:30 P.M. and gets out of bed at 7:15 A.M.

Bedtime = 10:30 P.M. = [(10 ∗ 60) + 30] −720 = [600 + 30] − 720 =
630 − 720 = −90 minutes

Time out of bed = 7:15 A.M. = (7 ∗ 60) + 15 = 420 + 15 = 435 minutes

Time in bed = Time out of bed − Bedtime = 435 − (−90) = 435 + 90 =
525 minutes

Expressed as hours, 525 minutes = 525/60 = 8.75 hours =
8 hours + 0.75 hours = 8 + (0.75 ∗ 60) = 8 hours, 45 minutes = 8:45

Calculating TST

1. Calculate the difference between "tried to go to sleep" and "finally woke at" in minutes.
2. Calculate sleep latency in minutes (if necessary).
3. Calculate wake after sleep onset (WASO), which is the sum of all awakenings in minutes.
4. TST = [(Difference between "finally woke at" and "tried to go to sleep at") – (sleep latency + WASO)]

For example, suppose the client in the previous example actually tried to go to sleep at 10:45 P.M., took 30 minutes to fall asleep, had three awakenings lasting a total of 1 hour and 10 minutes, and finally woke at 6:50 A.M.

First, convert "tried to go to sleep at" and "finally woke at" to minutes:

$$10:45 \text{ P.M.} = [(10 * 60) + 45] - 720 = [600 + 45] - 720 = 645 - 720 =$$
$$- 75 \text{ minutes (before midnight)}$$

$$6:50 \text{ A.M.} = (6 * 60) + 50 = 360 + 50 = 410 \text{ minutes (after midnight)}$$

Calculate the difference between "finally woke at" and "tried to go to sleep at" in minutes:

$$410 - (-75) = 410 + 75 = 485 \text{ minutes}$$

$$\text{Sleep latency} = 30 \text{ minutes}$$

$$\text{WASO} = 1:10 = (1 * 60) + 10 = 60 + 10 = 70 \text{ minutes}$$

$$\text{Sleep latency} + \text{WASO} = 30 \text{ minutes} + 70 \text{ minutes} = 100 \text{ minutes}$$

$$\text{TST} = [(\text{Difference between "finally woke at" and "tried to go to sleep at"}) -$$
$$(\text{sleep latency} + \text{sum of WASO})] = 485 \text{ minutes} - 100 \text{ minutes} = 385 \text{ minutes}$$

In hours and minutes the TST would be:

$$385 \text{ minutes} = 385/60 = 6.42 \text{ hours} = 6 \text{ hours} + 0.42 \text{ hours} =$$
$$6 \text{ hours} + (0.42 * 60) \text{ minutes} = 6 \text{ hours } 25 \text{ minutes} = 6:25$$

Calculating SE

1. Calculate TIB.
2. Calculate TST.
3. SE = (TST/TIB) * 100

In the example above, we determined that TIB = 525 minutes and TST = 385 minutes. Therefore:

$$SE = (TST/TIB) * 100 = (385/525) * 100 = 0.73 * 100 = 73\% \ SE$$

Calculating MST

1. Convert "bedtime" and "got out of bed at" to minutes.
2. Calculate the difference between "got out of bed at" and "bedtime."
3. Divide this difference by 2.
4. Subtract this number from "got out of bed at."
5. After calculating the weekly average, convert minutes back to hours.

In the example above, we previously determined that "bedtime" occurred at –90 minutes (i.e., 90 minutes before midnight, or 10:30 P.M.) and that "got out of bed at" occurred at 435 minutes (i.e., 435 minutes after midnight, or 7:15 A.M.). Further, we calculated that the difference between these two is 525 minutes.

Divide this difference by 2:

$$525/2 = 262.5 \ \text{minutes}$$

Subtract this number from "got out of bed at":

$$435 - 262.5 = 172.5 \ \text{minutes after midnight}$$

Convert back to hours and minutes:

$$172.5 \ \text{minutes} = 172.5/60 = 2.9 \ \text{hours} = 2 \ \text{hours} + 0.9 \ \text{hours} =$$
$$2 \ \text{hours} + (0.9 * 60) \ \text{minutes} = 2 \ \text{hours} + 54 \ \text{minutes} = 2{:}54$$

MST on this night is 2:54 A.M.

A Final Word

When calculating the average weekly values for TIB, TST, and MST, it is much easier to work in minutes and to convert back to hours at the end of the calculation. In other words, calculate each of these variables for each day in minutes. After averaging the minutes across the week, convert the average value back to hours and minutes. This will save spending a lot of time with your calculator!

A further potential advantage of completing the sleep diary is that the enhanced awareness arising from self-monitoring can have a therapeutic effect (Morin, 1993). Following several days of diary keeping clients can realize, from their written records, that they obtained more sleep than they initially thought. Thus they became less anxious about their sleep problem, which in turn creates a psychological state that is more conducive to sleep. Or through keeping the diary, clients realize that they sleep worse when their sleep schedule is irregular, which leads them to make a schedule adjustment, in turn improving sleep.

We ask clients to keep the sleep diary throughout the treatment sessions, and it is important to give them a rationale for this request—for example: "Maintaining a daily sleep diary is an important part of this program. We use the diary to plan and individualize the treatment just for you, and this is the way we monitor progress." Indeed, the daily diary is necessary for documenting the nature and severity of the initial sleep problem, assessing night-to-night variations in sleep patterns and identifying factors that contribute to improving or worsening sleep (we ask the client to make notes of these factors on the back of their diary or on a separate self-monitoring form), monitoring overall treatment progress, and evaluating progress with specific treatment modules.

It is difficult to conduct an effective treatment session when a client does not monitor his or her sleep or forgets to bring in the diary. Gently and briefly problem solve to maximize the chance that the diary will be completed in the coming week. If the client does not have the weekly sleep diary, we ask him or her to complete the diary for last night and then assess how typical this night was. This is a quick way to derive a proxy for the week of sleep. We do not recommend trying to reconstruct the entire week of sleep because people tend to not have accurate memories and the reconstruction process takes up a lot of time.

Watching the clock in an attempt to provide accurate times on the sleep diary should be discouraged. In fact, there is evidence indicating that clock watching contributes to increased anxiety and poorer ability to estimate sleep accurately (Tang, Schmidt, & Harvey, 2007). Instead, ask the client to base his or her sleep estimates on a best guess or a "felt sense." Only estimates are needed; absolute accuracy (which is impossible!) is not. Instead, place the emphasis on the daily recording.

To promote the completion of the sleep diary every morning, identify a time (breakfast) and location (kitchen) for completing the diary.

Early in each treatment session review the sleep diary by

- Checking the time the client went to bed for the 7 nights. How regular or irregular is the bedtime for the 7 days?
- Checking the time the client woke up for the 7 mornings. How regular or irregular is the wake time for the 7 days?

- Are there any long sleep onset latencies? How many? For how long?
- Are there any long awakenings after sleep onset? How many? For how long?
- Notice if the client is snoozing in the morning (i.e., staying in bed after wake-up time).
- Notice if the client wakes up during the night—how many times and for how long?
- Notice if there are naps.

This week-by-week sleep diary review, which we share with the client, is the basis for delivering many of the elements of TranS-C.

Functioning on the Six Sleep Health Dimensions

Achieving good sleep health is the central goal of TranS-C. We recommend using the daily sleep diary and the PROMIS scales to assess each client's functioning on the six dimensions of sleep health introduced in Chapter 1. The sleep diary in Figure 2.1 features a list of questions that illustrate these six dimensions. The last four items in the sleep diary in Figure 2.1 are the four key variables to be calculated by the clinician (see Box 2.1 for instructions). Rough estimates for these calculations are just fine.

- *Regularity.* Use the daily sleep diary to calculate the MST (i.e., midpoint time of the client's sleeping period). In Figure 2.1, the MST averaged across the week is 4:24 A.M. Observe the fluctuation around the midpoint for each night of the sleep diary. Reducing night-to-night fluctuation will be a treatment goal with this patient.

- *Satisfaction.* Use the daily sleep diary question on perceived sleep quality (question 11) or the sleep quality question on the PROMIS Sleep Disturbance scale. In Figure 2.1, the sleep quality ratings vary from night to night. As such, improving sleep quality will be a treatment goal when delivering TranS-C to this client.

- *Alertness.* Use the nap duration or number from the daily sleep diary (question 1) or the daytime sleepiness question on PROMIS Sleep-Related Impairment scale. The pattern of naps in Figure 2.1 is acceptable as the client is napping only 20 minutes before 3:00 P.M. This provides enough time for the client to rebuild the homeostatic pressure to sleep.

- *Timing.* Calculate the MST. Based on population-level data, we encourage the MST to fall within the range of 2:00 A.M. to 4:00 A.M. Most of the midpoints in Figure 2.1 are outside of this range.

My Sleep Diary

	Example 1/9/17	7/26/17	7/27/17	7/28/17	7/29/17	7/30/17	7/31/17	8/1/17
Date								
Day	Monday	Wednesday	Thursday	Friday	Saturday	Sunday	Monday	Tuesday
For which night's sleep?	Sunday	Tuesday	Wednesday	Thursday	Friday	Saturday	Sunday	Monday
1. Please list the time and length of naps you took yesterday.	11:30–11:45 P.M. 3–5 P.M.	0	20 min 2p.m.	0	0	20 min 1:00 p.m.	0	0
2a. How many drinks containing alcohol did you have yesterday?	2 drinks	0 drinks	0 drinks	0 drinks	0 drinks	0 drinks	0 drinks	0 drinks
2b. What time was your last alcoholic drink?	7:30 A.M. / (P.M.)	N/A A.M. / P.M.	N/A A.M. / P.M.	N/A A.M. / P.M.	N/A A.M. / P.M.	N/A A.M. / P.M.	N/A A.M. / P.M.	N/A A.M. / P.M.
3a. How many caffeinated drinks (coffee, tea, soda, energy drinks) did you have yesterday?	3 drinks	0 drinks	0 drinks	0 drinks	2 drinks	0 drinks	1 drinks	0 drinks

(continued)

FIGURE 2.1. Example of a completed sleep diary.

37

3b. What time was your last caffeinated drink?	8:00 (A.M.)/ P.M.	N/A A.M. / (P.M.)	N/A A.M. / (P.M.)	N/A A.M. / (P.M.)	N/A (A.M.) / P.M.	N/A A.M. / (P.M.)	N/A A.M. / P.M.
4. What time did you get into bed last night?	12:45 (A.M.)/ P.M.	1:30 (A.M.)/ P.M.	11:45 A.M. / (P.M.)	11:30 A.M. / (P.M.)	11:00 A.M. / (P.M.)	11:00 A.M. / (P.M.)	4:00 (A.M.)/ P.M.	10:30 A.M. / (P.M.)
5. What time did you try to go to sleep?	1:15 (A.M.)/ P.M.	1:30 (A.M.)/ P.M.	11:45 A.M. / (P.M.)	11:30 A.M. / (P.M.)	11:00 A.M. / (P.M.)	11:00 A.M. / (P.M.)	4:00 (A.M.)/ P.M.	11:00 A.M. / (P.M.)
6. How long did it take you to fall asleep?	__ hr(s) 30 min(s)	__ hr(s) 30 min(s)	__ hr(s) 30 min(s)	__ hr(s) 30 min(s)	__ hr(s) 0 min(s)	__ hr(s) 20 min(s)	__ hr(s) 20 min(s)	__ hr(s) 30 min(s)
7. How many times did you wake up, not counting your final awakening?	2 times	2 times	2 times	1 times	0 times	2 times	0 times	2 times
8. For how long did each awakening last?	1st awakening __ hr(s) 30 min(s) / 2nd awakening 1 hr(s) 30 min(s) / 3rd awakening __ hr(s) __ min(s)	1st awakening __ hr(s) 30 min(s) / 2nd awakening __ hr(s) 30 min(s) / 3rd awakening __ hr(s) __ min(s)	1st awakening 3 hr(s) __ min(s) / 2nd awakening 1 hr(s) __ min(s) / 3rd awakening __ hr(s) __ min(s)	1st awakening 3 hr(s) __ min(s) / 2nd awakening __ hr(s) __ min(s) / 3rd awakening __ hr(s) __ min(s)	1st awakening __ hr(s) __ min(s) / 2nd awakening __ hr(s) __ min(s) / 3rd awakening __ hr(s) __ min(s)	1st awakening __ hr(s) 30 min(s) / 2nd awakening __ hr(s) 30 min(s) / 3rd awakening __ hr(s) __ min(s)	1st awakening __ hr(s) 20 min(s) / 2nd awakening __ hr(s) 20 min(s) / 3rd awakening __ hr(s) __ min(s)	1st awakening __ hr(s) 20 min(s) / 2nd awakening __ hr(s) 20 min(s) / 3rd awakening __ hr(s) __ min(s)

(continued)

FIGURE 2.1. *(continued)*

9. What time was your final awakening?	7:45 (A.M.) / P.M.	9:30 (A.M.) / P.M.	8:00 (A.M.) / P.M.	7:00 (A.M.) / P.M.	8:00 (A.M.) / P.M.	8:00 (A.M.) / P.M.	7:30 (A.M.) / P.M.	7:40 (A.M.) / P.M.
10. What time did you get out of bed for the day?	7:45 (A.M.) / P.M.	9:30 (A.M.) / P.M.	11:00 (A.M.) / P.M.	7:00 (A.M.) / P.M.	8:30 (A.M.) / P.M.	9:00 (A.M.) / P.M.	7:30 (A.M.) / P.M.	8:00 (A.M.) / P.M.
11. How would you rate the quality of your sleep last night? 1 2 3 4 5 6 7 Poor Sleep Quality — Excellent Sleep Quality	1 (poor)	5	2	3	7	4	5	4

TO BE COMPLETED BY CLINICIAN

Time in Bed (TIB)		8 hrs 00 min	11 hrs 15 min	7 hrs 30 min	9 hrs 30 min	10 hrs 00 min	3 hrs 30 min	9 hrs 30 min
Total Sleep Time (TST)		6 hrs 30 min	3 hrs 45 min	4 hrs 00 min	9 hrs 00 min	7 hrs 40 min	3 hrs 10 min	7 hrs 30 min
Sleep Efficiency (SE)		81%	33%	53%	95%	77%	90%	79%
Midsleep Time (MST)		5:30 A.M.	5:24 A.M.	3:15 A.M.	3:45 A.M.	4:00 A.M.	5:45 A.M.	3:15 A.M.

Weekly Average Values
TIB: 8 hrs 28 min
TST: 5 hrs 56 min
SE: 72.7%
MST: 4:24 A.M.

39

FIGURE 2.1. (continued)

• *Efficiency.* Use the calculated sleep efficiency or the reported total wake time based on the daily sleep diary. As evident in Figure 2.1, sleep efficiency varies from 33 to 95%. The intervention to improve sleep efficiency is usually needed when the average sleep efficiency is below 85% (the cutoff is adapted to 80% for older adults).

• *Duration.* Use the mean TST based on the daily sleep diary. In Figure 2.1, the TST varies from around 3 hours per night up to 9 hours per night. The recommended sleep duration for adults is 7–8 hours per night.

Progress on improving each of these dimensions can be tracked with the daily sleep diary during the course of treatment.

Assessments for the TranS-C Modules

Table 2.1 summarizes the assessments we recommend for each of the TranS-C modules. Most of the TranS-C modules can be assessed from the sleep diary or from the information collected during the case formulation described in Chapter 3 (i.e., Cross-Cutting Module 1). However, there are a few exceptions.

First, the two assessments of Core Module 2 on improving daytime functioning are designed to distinguish between sleepiness and fatigue. This is an important distinction. Sleepiness refers to the propensity to fall asleep unintentionally or the struggle to remain awake. Fatigue refers to low physical or mental energy levels, often equated with tiredness or weariness. We propose using the Epworth Sleepiness Scale (Johns, 1991) for the former assessment and the Fatigue Severity Scale (Krupp, LaRocca, Muir-Nash, & Steinberg, 1989) for the latter assessment. Note that clients who meet criteria for insomnia are more likely to experience fatigue, but are typically not sleepy (Stepanski, Zorick, Roehrs, Young, & Roth, 1988).

Second, the Dysfunctional Beliefs and Attitudes about Sleep scale (DBAS; Morin, 1993) is used to assess unhelpful beliefs about sleep, needed for Core Module 3. The DBAS is a 30-item self-report scale that examines a broad range of sleep-related cognitions (beliefs, attitudes, expectations, and attributions) that are proposed to maintain insomnia. They can be grouped into four areas: (1) sleep expectations, (2) causal attributions of insomnia, (3) perceived consequences of insomnia, and (4) worry/helplessness about insomnia. A higher score reflects more dysfunctional beliefs. A 16-item short version has also been validated (Espie, Inglis, Harvey, & Tessier, 2000). In addition, a 10-item child version has been developed (Blunden, Gregory, & Crawford, 2013; Gregory, Cox, Crawford, Holland, & Harvey, 2009).

TABLE 2.1. Assessment of the TranS-C Modules

Common Trans-C problems	Assessment measure	No. of items	Format
Core Module 1, Part A: Establishing regular sleep–wake times	Daily sleep diary		
Core Module 1, Part B: Learning a wind-down routine	Cross-Cutting Module 1		
Core Module 1, Part C: Learning a wake-up routine	Cross-Cutting Module 1		
Core Module 2: Improving daytime functioning	Epworth Sleepiness Scale	8	4-point scale (0 = "no chance," 3 = "high chance")
	Fatigue Severity Scale	9	7-point scale (1 = "strongly disagree," 7 = "strongly agree")
Core Module 3: Correcting unhelpful sleep-related beliefs	Dysfunctional Beliefs and Attitudes about Sleep scale	30 or 16	11-point scale (0 = "strongly disagree," 10 = "strongly agree")
Optional Module 1: Improving sleep efficiency	Daily sleep diary		
Optional Module 2: Reducing time in bed	Daily sleep diary		
Optional Module 3: Dealing with delayed or advanced phase	Daily sleep diary		
Optional Module 4: Reducing sleep-related worry/vigilance	Anxiety and Preoccupation about Sleep Questionnaire	10	10-point scale (1 = "not true," 10 = "very true")
Optional Module 5: Promoting compliance with the CPAP machine/exposure therapy for claustrophobic reactions to the CPAP	CPAP Habit Index	5	5-point scale (1–5 anchors change depending on the subscale)
	Attitudes toward CPAP Use Questionnaire	34	5-point scale (1 = "strongly agree," 5 = "strongly disagree")
Optional Module 6: Negotiating sleep in a complicated environment	Cross-Cutting Module 1		
Optional Module 7: Reducing nightmares	Daily sleep diary		

Third, the Anxiety and Preoccupation about Sleep Questionnaire (APSQ; Jansson-Fröjmark, Harvey, Lundh, Norell-Clarke, & Linton, 2011; Tang & Harvey, 2004) is a brief assessment of the extent to which people worry about their sleep and assists in determining the need for Optional Module 4, which addresses sleep-related worry and vigilance. The APSQ is sensitive to the effects of treatment (Harvey, Sharpley, Ree, Stinson, & Clark, 2007).

Fourth, we determine the need for Optional Module 5, which addresses treatment adherence for sleep apnea, with the CPAP Habit Index (CHI; Broström et al., 2014), which is a brief assessment of adherence to CPAP. Also, the longer and more detailed Attitudes toward CPAP Use Questionnaire (Stepnowsky, Marler, & Ancoli-Israel, 2002) can be very helpful. It includes an assessment of self-efficacy (5 items; e.g., "I am confident I can use CPAP regularly"), outcome expectations (2 items; e.g., "How important do you believe regular use of CPAP is for controlling your sleep apnea?"), social support (9 items; e.g., "I have people in my life who will support me in using CPAP regularly"), and knowledge (12 items; e.g., "One of the main symptoms of sleep apnea is excessive daytime sleepiness").

Assessment of Common Sleep Disorders

Structured Interview to Screen for Sleep Disorders

The Duke Structured Interview for Sleep Disorders (DSISD) is a structured series of questions that helps the clinician to efficiently establish sleep disorder diagnoses according to the *Diagnostic and Statistical Manual of Mental Disorders* (DSM-5; American Psychiatric Association, 2013) and the *International Classification of Sleep Disorders* (ICSD-3; American Academy of Sleep Medicine, 2014). Each section of the interview starts with a screening question. If this is endorsed, a series of follow-up questions are asked. If the screening question is not endorsed, the follow-up questions are skipped, and the assessor moves to the screening question in the next category. The DSISD is divided into three sections: insomnia diagnoses, other sleep disorders (e.g., dyssomnia), and sleep disorders associated with excessive daytime sleepiness.

Additional Questionnaire Assessments

We screen for obstructive sleep apnea (OSA) and restless leg syndrome (RLS) by supplementing the proposed DUKE assessment with the STOP-Bang questionnaire (Farney, Walker, Farney, Snow, & Walker, 2011), an 8-item screen for OSA, and the International Restless Legs Syndrome Study Group (IRLSSG) rating scale (Walters et al., 2003), is a 10-item screen for RLS. Both measures are validated, but there are limitations. First, self-report measures of these disorders are limited in their sensitivity to detect these disorders. Individuals who screen positively should be referred to their primary care provider for consideration of a full gold-standard evaluation and treatment. Second, the STOP-Bang requires measurements of neck size, weight, and height. Clients are likely to need assistance to obtain these measurements. Clients with OSA and RLS are not excluded from TranS-C, as they often also have one or more sleep and circadian problems that can be addressed with this intervention.

Sleep Disorders Addressed by TranS-C

Insomnia Disorder

Insomnia disorder consists of ongoing problems with getting to sleep, staying asleep, or waking up too early, as well as problems with daytime functioning. An important aspect of insomnia is that patients must be providing themselves sufficient opportunity to get enough sleep.

Various quantitative criteria for insomnia have been offered. DSM-5 states that the insomnia must be present for "at least 3 nights" per week for "at least 3 months"(American Psychiatric Association, 2013, p. 362). Lichstein, Durrence, Taylor, Bush, and Riedel (2003) require that self-reported sleep onset latency (SOL) or wakefulness after sleep onset (WASO) must be equal to or longer than 31 minutes for at least 3 nights per week over a period of at least 6 months. Readers are also referred to Buysse et al. (2006), who offer additional quantitative criteria for insomnia.

Insomnia *disorder* requires the presence of nighttime insomnia *symptoms,* but these symptoms may also be present in a range of other sleep disorders. For example, insomnia symptoms are listed as a feature of various sleep-related breathing disorders, circadian rhythm disorders, and sleep-related movement disorders, as well as the parasomnias (e.g., nightmare disorder and sleep-related breathing disorder). Such symptoms can arise, at least in part, from the precipitating factors that are also a feature of the insomnia disorders (e.g., hyperarousal, conditioning). The distinction between insomnia disorder and other sleep disorders rests on the presence of other symptoms and findings. For instance, insomnia symptoms in sleep apnea are accompanied by repeated breathing pauses observed during a sleep study, and insomnia symptoms with RLS are accompanied by other motor symptoms. Of course, this common overlap in symptoms is part of the rationale for TranS-C.

The TranS-C modules that are likely to be most relevant for clients who meet the diagnostic criteria for insomnia are the four core modules and Optional Modules 1 and 4.

Too Much Time in Bed

Many clients, particularly those with a mental illness, spend too much time in bed, a sleep problem that has been attributed to a "lack of interest, withdrawal, decreased energy . . . rather than true sleep propensity" (Nofzinger et al., 1991, p. 1177) or to "anergia" without objective daytime sleepiness (Billiard, Dolenc, Aldaz, Ondze, & Besset, 1994).

It is important to distinguish among three different sleep problems: *narcolepsy, hypersomnolence disorder, and too much time in bed*. See Table 2.2 for these distinctions. If narcolepsy or hypersomnolence disorder are suspected, the client should be referred to a physician. More information on these disorders is provided in the section "Sleep Disorders to Refer to a Sleep Specialist." If spending too much time in bed is suspected, the client can be treated by TranS-C (particularly Optional Module 2).

TABLE 2.2. Distinctions between Narcolepsy, Hypersomnolence Disorder, and Too Much Time in Bed

	Narcolepsy	Hypersomnolence disorder	Too much TIB
Daytime sleepiness	Severe (irrepressible need to sleep, inadvertent sleep episodes, naps)	Severe (naps, inadvertent sleep episodes)	Less severe; tiredness > sleepiness (voluntary naps)
MSLT (if available)	Short SOL (<8 minutes) and REM at sleep onset	Short SOL (<8 minutes)	Normal to borderline short SOL (8–10 minutes)
Too much time in bed	Normal	Long or normal	Long
Sleep continuity	Frequent brief awakenings	High	Low
Wakefulness in bed	Frequent brief awakenings	Low	High
Sleep inertia	Yes	Yes	Yes
Motivation for daytime activity	Higher	Higher	Lower
Desire for daytime sleep	Low (seek to avoid)	Low (seek to avoid)	High (perceive few or no behavioral alternatives)

Note. SOL, Sleep onset latency; REM, rapid-eye-movement sleep; TIB, time in bed; MSLT, multiple sleep latency test.

Circadian Rhythm Disorders

These disorders are characterized by an atypical timing of sleep, reflecting a mismatch between the client's sleep–wake rhythm and that required by his or her lifestyle or employment. DSM-5 requires that "the sleep disruption leads to excessive sleepiness or insomnia or both" (American Psychiatric Association, 2013, p. 390) and describes four subtypes that TranS-C addresses. The *delayed sleep phase type* involves not being able to fall asleep until the early hours in the morning and sleeping well into the next day. The *advanced sleep phase type* involves falling asleep early and waking up early. The *irregular sleep–wake type* involves an irregular 24-hour sleep–wake pattern. In the *non-24-hour sleep–wake type,* the sleep and wake pattern is not associated with the conventional 24-hour period and wake and sleep times tend to move later each day. When the latter pattern is due to blindness, we recommend the treatment approaches described by Sack and colleagues (Sack, Brandes, Kendall, & Lewy, 2000; Sack & Lewy, 2001) instead of TranS-C.

The TranS-C modules that are likely to be most relevant to clients who meet the diagnostic criteria for delayed and advanced phase circadian rhythm disorders are the four core modules and Optional Module 3. For the irregular sleep–wake type, Core Module 1 is recommended.

Sleep Disorders to Refer to a Sleep Specialist

Sleep Apnea

Sleep apnea is characterized by repeated breathing pauses or shallow breathing during sleep. These episodes, which may occur hundreds of times per night, lead to repeated episodes of reduced blood oxygen saturation levels ("desaturations"), transient arousals, and more prolonged awakenings. In obstructive sleep apnea (OSA), apnea episodes are caused by a collapse of the airway during inspiration; in central sleep apnea (CSA), the effort to breathe is transiently suspended by brain signals. Nighttime symptoms of sleep apnea can include snoring, pauses in breathing during sleep, shortness of breath during sleep, choking during sleep, awakening with a gasp or snort, headaches on waking, or difficulty drawing breath or breathlessness on waking. Common daytime symptoms include sleepiness, fatigue, and unrefreshing sleep. Overnight polysomnographic testing, described in a later section, provides an objective assessment of sleep apnea.

The most common treatment for sleep apnea is CPAP, in which a small compressor delivers pressurized air through a nasal–oral mask to maintain the patency of the airway during sleep. Other treatments include oral appliances, surgery, and upper airway stimulation devices.

There is evidence that clients with sleep apnea benefit from CBT-I (Wu et al., 2015), and they often exhibit the sleep and circadian problems covered by TranS-C. As such, while referring clients suspected of sleep apnea for evaluation by a sleep specialist is warranted, we also include these clients in TranS-C.

Restless Leg Syndrome

The hallmark symptom of RLS is an impulse to move the limbs (usually the legs). This urge may be accompanied by restlessness or unpleasant sensations in the extremities, often described as "creepy-crawly" feelings under the skin. Although symptoms in the legs are most common, they may also occur in the arms or other body parts. The symptoms have a circadian pattern, increasing in the evening hours, peaking in the early night, and subsiding by morning. Symptoms typically start or get worse when resting, relaxing, or first going to bed, and are promptly relieved by movement, such as walking, tapping, or stretching. For some RLS clients the discomfort is sufficient enough to interfere with falling asleep. Clients with suspected RLS should be referred to their physician for further evaluation. A physician will ensure that RLS is distinguished from akathisia secondary to neuroleptics use, or determine whether RLS may have been precipitated by the use of other psychiatric medications.

Typical treatments for RLS include dopamine agonist drugs, such as pramipexole or ropinirole; gabapentin; iron supplementation; benzodiazepines; and in some cases, low doses of opiate medications.

Periodic Limb Movement Disorder (PLMD)

The hallmark feature of periodic limb movement disorder (PLMD) is repetitive episodes of limb movements, usually in the legs, during sleep. The movements are associated with a partial or full awakening. Those affected may have hundreds of movements or brisk extensions of the feet during the night. It is not uncommon for these movements to be associated with a hundred or more brief arousals. On occasion a limb movement will produce a shift to a full awakening. However, typically the client is not aware of the limb movements. The clinician will need to infer their presence from the bed partner's report, for example, that the client is a "restless sleeper" or "kicks" during the night. Overnight polysomnographic testing, conducted by a sleep specialist, provides objective evidence of PLMD. Most clients with RLS also have PLMD. This is important as these clients can benefit from RLS-specific treatments.

There is evidence that clients with PLMD benefit from CBT-I (Wu et al., 2015), and they often exhibit the sleep and circadian problems covered by TranS-C. As such, while it is important to refer clients suspected of PLMD for evaluation by a sleep specialist, we also include these clients in TranS-C.

Narcolepsy

The core symptom of narcolepsy is a persistent struggle to maintain alertness and wakefulness during the day. This sleepiness may manifest as inadvertent sleep episodes, naps, or episodes of "automatic behavior" while sleepy. Perhaps surprisingly, many clients with narcolepsy also complain of frequent brief awakenings at night. Thus, narcolepsy may be considered a disorder of sleep–wake state control, with difficulty sustaining wakefulness *and* difficulty maintaining sleep. The cause of narcolepsy is a loss of neurons containing the neurotransmitter orexin (also called hypocretin), whose function is to stabilize the activity of wake-promoting neurons in the brain stem. A subset of clients with narcolepsy also have cataplexy, which is a sudden loss of muscle tone. Clients with narcolepsy may have two other symptoms that occur at sleep–wake or wake–sleep transitions: sleep paralysis, which is an inability to move despite feeling awake, and sleep-related auditory, visual, or tactile hallucinations. Cataplexy, sleep paralysis, and sleep-related hallucinations can all be thought of as other indicators of sleep–wake state instability. Specifically, these symptoms represent admixtures of rapid-eye-movement (REM) sleep (skeletal muscle paralysis, vivid sensory experiences) and wakefulness. Not surprisingly, the symptoms of narcolepsy are sometimes mistaken for those of a psychiatric disorder, given features such as strong emotion triggers and hallucinatory experiences. Clients with suspected narcolepsy should be referred to a medically trained sleep specialist, who may conduct a thorough assessment, including a clinical evaluation, overnight polysomnogram, and a multiple sleep latency test (described in the section on additional assessments). Virtually all clients with narcolepsy are treated with stimulant medications.

Hypersomnolence Disorder

A diagnosis of hypersomnolence disorder is given when a client experiences difficulty staying alert during the day despite sleeping 7 or more hours each night. The client might also involuntarily fall asleep during the day and have difficulty waking in the morning or after a nap. Unlike clients with narcolepsy, those with hypersomnolence disorder do not have cataplexy, nor are sleep paralysis or sleep-related hallucinations common. While many individuals with narcolepsy report that short naps restore alertness, those with hypersomnolence disorder typically report that longer naps are followed by sleep inertia and persistent sleepiness. Orexin levels are normal in the brains of clients with hypersomnolence disorder, although recent evidence suggests that they may have elevated levels of endogenous benzodiazepine-like neurochemicals. Clients with this disorder should also receive an evaluation by a sleep specialist, and most are treated with stimulant medications.

Parasomnias

This cluster of disorders includes sleep walking and sleep terrors, which involve intense fear and screaming. Clients often cannot recall the episodes. Parasomnias usually occur during the first third of the night. Again, clients with this presentation should be referred to their physician for consideration of a full evaluation and treatment (American Psychiatric Association, 2013).

REM Sleep Behavior Disorder

This disorder is characterized by sounds or speech and movement during sleep. Clients may act as if they are being attacked or trying to escape. These behaviors can result in injury. However, clients are immediately alert when awakened.

Additional Assessments of Sleep

Polysomnography

Polysomnography (PSG) is an overnight "sleep study." The procedures in PSG are adapted from those of electroencephalography (EEG) and other electrophysiological techniques. In PSG, a client is monitored overnight to derive information about sleep, sleep stages, and other physiological events during sleep, such as apnea, blood oxygen desaturation, and abnormal heart rhythms. PSG involves placing electrodes on specific sites on the scalp to measure EEG, on the chin to measure electromyographic (EMG) signals, and beside the eyes to measure electro-oculographic (EOG) signals. The EEG is used to classify sleep into stages (stage W [wake] and stages N1–N3 [non-REM]). The EMG and EOG are needed to score rapid eye movements (stage R [REM]). During REM there is a loss of muscle tone and circular rhythmic eye movements. Measures of respiration (oral–nasal air flow, respiratory effort in the chest and abdomen, oxygen saturation, electrocardiogram) are used to evaluate the presence of sleep apnea. Anterior tibialis EMG electrodes are added to the lower legs to evaluate periodic limb movements during sleep. PSG is typically conducted in a sleep laboratory but is occasionally completed at home. Home sleep apnea testing is a simplified version of PSG that includes only respiratory measures to identify sleep apnea. In most cases, home sleep apnea testing does not include data on sleep or sleep stages.

PSG is typically not recommended for the routine evaluation of insomnia, circadian rhythm sleep–wake disorders, or RLS (e.g., Kushida et al., 2005; Littner et al., 2003). However, it is important to refer clients to a sleep specialist for clinical evaluation and PSG when other sleep disorders are suspected, including sleep apnea, narcolepsy, PLMD, and parasomnias. A referral to a sleep specialist may also be warranted if the client does not respond to TranS-C. In the latter case, a comorbid sleep disorder may be present but covert, especially when there is no bed partner who may observe or complain about the symptoms. The major limitations of PSG include its relatively high cost and inconvenience.

Simpler and cheaper methods are being developed. For example, Apnea-Link Plus is a home monitoring device consisting of oral–nasal thermistors, fingertip oximetry, and piezoelectric respirator-effort belts to screen for sleep apnea. This device shows a high correlation (> .85) with standard PSG (Clark, Crabbe, Aziz, Reddy, & Greenstone, 2009; Erman, Stewart, & Einhorn, 2007; Nigro, Dibur, Aimaretti, González, & Rhodius, 2011; Oktay et al., 2011; Ragette, Wang, Weinreich, & Teschler, 2010).

Multiple Sleep Latency Test

The multiple sleep latency test (MSLT) is an objective assessment of excessive daytime sleepiness and is used to diagnose narcolepsy. Clients are typically given five 20-minute nap opportunities at 2-hour intervals during one day. The time taken to fall asleep is the index of sleepiness, and the stages of sleep during the nap are scored. If the client falls asleep in less than 8 minutes and REM sleep is observed in two or more naps, a diagnosis of narcolepsy is considered (REM sleep typically occurs after 70–90 minutes of sleeping). The client is awakened after sleeping for 15 minutes. If the client does not fall asleep within 20 minutes, the test ends.

Summary

In summary, the assessments described in this chapter represent a multimethod approach that, at minimum, includes clinical and semistructured interviews, questionnaires, and daily monitoring with the sleep diary. The goal is to establish the suitability of the client for TranS-C, to formulate a diagnosis, and to begin devising the treatment plan.

CHAPTER 3

TranS-C Cross-Cutting Modules

The four cross-cutting modules—Case Formulation, Sleep and Circadian Education, Behavior Change and Motivation, and Goal Setting—are *typically* introduced in the first treatment session once the assessment phase has been completed. Thereafter they become *rolling interventions,* which means that session-by-session we embrace opportunities that arise to continue to develop the case formulation and to remind the client of the key sleep and circadian education points. We also flexibly interweave the tools of behavior change and evaluate the client's goals, setting new goals as needed. We suggest that these modules be *typically* introduced in the first treatment session because the pace at which each client will prefer to move through the session material can vary substantially. It is critical to be sensitive to whether the client has had enough time to fully grasp all aspects of each module before moving on. Ask questions on a regular basis to check the client's understanding of the session content and to determine whether the pace is appropriate.

Cross-Cutting Module 1: Case Formulation

In this module, the therapist becomes acquainted with the client and reviews information about his or her sleep experiences and problems before beginning the actual intervention. Note that we don't use the term "case formulation" when speaking with a client; we avoid jargon and use everyday language.

Presession Preparation

In some contexts (e.g., if you are working at a sleep specialty clinic), you may already have a copy of the client's completed daily sleep diary. If so, calculate the sleep parameters of interest (typically TIB, TST, SOL, WASO, and SE), and review the discussion in Chapter 2 on the most important aspects of the sleep diary to pay attention to, particularly noting which of the six dimensions of sleep health the client can improve. If you don't have the client's sleep diary, we recommend asking him or her to bring the diary to this session to be reviewed together, or teach the client how to fill in the sleep diary and ask him or her to complete it over the coming week, as described in Chapter 2 (see Appendix 13 for a blank sleep diary and instructions). Once you have the information from the sleep diary in hand, you will combine the information you glean from it into the formulation, as we illustrate in the "Combining Functional Analysis and Assessment" section.

Also, read through any assessment or referral materials you have and make a list of potential maintaining processes. If you get stuck during the case formulation, you can use this summary to engage in appropriate prompting. For some clients it can be helpful to refer directly to the responses on questionnaires completed during the assessment (e.g., the client can be asked to elaborate on his or her answers). Also be aware that many of the processes or behaviors are so habitual or automatic that they may not be consciously aware of them.

In the Session

Based on the approach to case formulation developed by David M. Clark and Anke Ehlers for anxiety disorders (e.g., Clark et al., 2006; Ehlers et al., 2003), we first give the client a rationale for the treatment. For example:

> "I'd like to begin by getting a very detailed picture of your experience of sleep. This will help us plan our sessions together. The way we do this is for us to identify together a recent typical night . . . I'll ask you lots of questions about this night so that I can get a sense of what is going on. This will help us develop a plan for our sessions together. It's like a fingerprint, everyone's is a bit different, so the treatment needs to be a bit different for each person. How does that sound?"

The next step is to work with the client to choose a *very specific, typical,* and *recent* example of a night of sleep during which the problem was evident. This example will then be used to conduct a functional analysis of the specific sleep episode.

- A *very specific* episode is a situation that happened on one particular day (e.g., last night). For example, a 17-year-old client, who selected Monday night, explained, "I had a terrible night. I was worried about college applications. I couldn't get to sleep for a while, and then I kept waking up." We recommend against basing the functional analysis on the client's sleep in general because it is difficult to average across a whole week and important details are missed.
- Check to what extent the selected night is *typical*. Sometimes it becomes obvious part of the way into the discussion that the night was not typical, for example, the client had food poisoning. At that point we recommend stopping and starting again with a typical night. That's why we keep multiple copies of the Personalized Case Conceptualization Form close by (see Appendix 3). It is better to spend precious session time on a truly typical night when the sleep problem is evident.
- Choosing a *recent* example is helpful because the client will have a clear memory of the episode.

Then we spend a few minutes asking the client information questions to start to get an idea of the context around the episode being discussed. For example, briefly ask about the preceding day and evening to determine whether anything happened that might have had a bearing on the sleep difficulty experienced that night. For example, having "a big fight with my husband" just before bedtime will likely affect the sleep obtained that night.

Then use the Personalized Case Conceptualization Form to elicit sleep-related behaviors, thoughts, feelings, and consequences at bedtime, during the night, on waking, and during the day. Use guided discovery to complete the blanks on the form, working across the rows on the form instead of down the page. That is, ask about behaviors, thoughts, and feelings for "At Bedtime," before moving to "In the Night." For the "During the Day" row, try to keep the questions focused on sleep—For example: "Did you think much about sleep in the day?"; "Did you have any sleep-related feelings in the day?"; "Did you do anything differently because you didn't sleep well the night before?"; or "Did you do anything in an attempt to help you sleep well tonight?" An example of the outcome of the process for an adolescent female client is presented in Box 3.1, and examples of questions to help complete the formulation are presented in Box 3.2.

Focus on Modifiable Factors

This process will uncover several modifiable behaviors and thoughts that become part of the road map for TranS-C. For example, for the case presented

BOX 3.1. An Example of a Functional Analysis Used
toward the Case Formulation for a 14-Year-Old Female

	What I was doing	What I was thinking	What I was feeling
At bedtime	• Brushed teeth • Got into bed • Looked at phone • Texted with boyfriend and got into a fight • Texted with friend about school project	• I'm so tired. • What's going on with my boyfriend? Is he about to break up with me? • I have so much more work to do on this project. I'm never going to finish in time.	• Exhausted • Annoyed • Angry • Overwhelmed • Stressed

Consequence: I lay awake thinking about my boyfriend and school stuff. I couldn't fall asleep for hours.

In the night	• I didn't wake up.		

Consequence: N/A

On waking	• I stayed in bed after the alarm went off, snoozing.	• I'm too tired to get up. • I don't want to go to school. • I don't think I can face classes or my boyfriend.	• Sad • Anxious • Tired

Consequence: Late for school. Had to get dressed quickly. No time for breakfast. Fought with my mom.

During the day	• Drank coke. • Was drowsy in class. • Napped after school.	• This class is so boring. I can't make sense of what is going on. • I can't wait to get home and sleep.	• Tired • Sad

Consequence: I couldn't concentrate in class. I'm already behind at school. Coke and napping might have made it harder to sleep the next night.

BOX 3.2. Helpful Questions to Ask
during the Functional Analysis

For identifying behaviors . . .

- "Take me through what you were doing step-by-step as you were getting ready for bed/as you woke in the night/from the moment you woke up in the morning/as the next day unfolded."
- "Is there anything you were doing to try to ensure you get to sleep/ perform well during the day?"

For identifying negative thoughts . . .

- "What went through your mind/what were you thinking before getting into bed/as you got into bed/on waking/as you got ready for the day, and as you noticed you weren't getting to sleep/weren't performing well?"
- "What was the worst you thought could happen?"
- "What would that mean? What would be so bad about that?"

For identifying feelings . . .

- "What were you feeling as all of this was unfolding?"
- "When you are afraid that _____ might happen, what did you notice happening in your body? What sensations did you experience?"
- "How about your energy level? Were you feeling tired or energetic?"

Drawing out the consequences . . .

- "Were there any consequences of these emotions for how the rest of your day went?/for getting back to sleep?"
- "Given all of this—these thoughts [name some], these feelings [name some], what was the consequence of all of this?"

For during the day . . .

- "Did you think much about sleep in the day?"
- "Did you have any sleep-related feelings in the day?"
- "Did you do anything differently that day because you didn't sleep well or to help you sleep well tonight?"

in Box 3.1 the possible modifiable maintaining behaviors and cognitions include: texting in bed, worrying about her boyfriend and school, staying in bed snoozing after the alarm rang, not eating breakfast, drinking cola while at school, and napping after school. It is easy to see how each of these factors contribute to the sleep problem. Texting in bed contributed to worrying, making it hard to get to sleep. Staying in bed snoozing contributed to not eating breakfast, which probably contributes to feeling drowsy in class and finding it hard to follow the content of the class. Drinking cola during the day at school can contribute to difficulties getting to sleep the next night. Napping in the afternoon after school discharges the homeostatic pressure to sleep, which can make it difficult to get to sleep and stay asleep the next night.

It's worth pointing out that there are typically a confluence of multiple contributors (5 to 10) to most sleep problems. Some of these contributors are modifiable, while others are not. In TranS-C, we focus on the modifiable factors. There will often be nonmodifiable factors present too. For example, for an adolescent client who reported feeling lethargic during the day, the factors that we uncovered include:

- The teen has several hours of homework to complete each night.
- The teen drinks a caffeinated energy drink while doing her homework.
- The teen watches several episodes of her favorite show and texts with friends before going to sleep at 1:00 A.M.
- The teen's alarm clock goes off at 6:00 A.M. Then she snoozes from 6:15 A.M. to 7:00 A.M.
- The teen's school starts at 7:30 A.M.
- The teen's teacher often shows films in a darkened classroom.
- The teen has to sit at a desk for most of the school day and has limited opportunities to move around.

The therapist accepted—and helped the teen to accept—that some of these factors cannot be easily changed, such as the amount of assigned homework, the school start time, a darkened classroom, and limited activity during the school day. Do not spend too much time discussing these factors. Instead, focus your discussion on the factors that are modifiable, namely, caffeine intake, nighttime technology use, and the snoozing habit.

The Final Stage of Case Formulation

This final stage of case formulation—arguably the most important part—can be easily forgotten by therapists. There are two steps, as follows.

Step 1: Introduce the Cognitive-Behavioral Model

Use the client's completed Personalized Case Conceptualization Form to intro-duce the cognitive-behavioral model. For example, you could say:

> "OK, this has been very helpful . . . This is very similar to what we often find [normalizing] . . . These kinds of thoughts [name some from the completed form] and these kinds of behaviors [name some] seem to lead to these kinds of feelings. And together, the behaviors, thoughts, and feel-ings make it difficult to fall sleep/wake up/cope during the day. On top of that, these kinds of thoughts [name some] and feelings [name some] can contribute to anxiety and worry."

Then pause and ask for the client's feedback as to whether or not this formula-tion makes sense. Use this feedback to make any modifications. Be aware that jargon can creep into your attempt to introduce the model. Box 3.3 offers some suggestions for simple everyday language to use.

BOX 3.3. Using Accessible Language in Summarizing the Case Conceptualization

Less inspiring and accessible phrases:

- "The reason we do this exercise is to show the effects your behaviors, thoughts, and feelings have on your sleep."
- "We are going to target these [behaviors/thoughts] in treatment."

More inspiring and accessible phrases:

- "Thank you for sharing with me—this is really very interesting and helpful and will help us as we plan the treatment."
- "What do you notice? What stands out to you?"
- "I'm struck by the way your [behaviors/thoughts] contribute to [con-sequences]. What do you make of that?"
- "The good news is we can do experiments to see what effect adjust-ing these [behaviors/thoughts] can have on your sleep. Would running some experiments together be of interest to you?"
- "Given what we're seeing here, I think there's a lot we can do together to make changes for the better. How does that sound?"

Step 2: Ask for the Client's Ideas for Ways to Intervene

For example, ask, "Given this, what do you think we should target in the sessions we have together to stop and reverse the vicious cycle?" Many clients are not able to come up with ways to intervene, so the therapist should help them by saying something like:

> "I suggest that one of our targets be these thoughts [name them]. If we can change them, we can change your feelings [point to the relevant parts of the completed form]. This alone will be very helpful for getting back to sleep. In addition, we'll also look at some of the behaviors that seem to be contributing too. How do you feel about those ideas?"

The message we want to convey is that a change in one or more parts of the vicious cycle will shift the system. In other words, this process provides a rationale for treatment and gives a sense of hope (and a reason to return for Session 2!).

We also introduce the possibility of completing behavioral experiments together.

> "If you are interested, we might set up some experiments to double check whether the things you are doing to cope right now are helpful or not. Sometimes we discover that they are feeding into the vicious cycle. Other times we find that the coping strategies are working well."

Following a similar process for a typical "good night" is also illuminating for clients with night-to-night variability in their sleep. We follow this process for a typical day following both poor and good nights, which can be helpful for discovering daytime maintaining processes.

As pointed out earlier in this chapter, the case formulation is initially completed after the assessment phase is conducted. However, further functional analysis, which can lead to an improved case formulation, should be provided in subsequent sessions as needed. For example, in future sessions, it is common for clients to report that they experienced a bad night of sleep without understanding why. This sense of loss of control of sleep is common and contributes to anxiety. In these circumstances it is very helpful to review the episode in detail by mapping out the vicious cycle on a blank sheet of paper, showing how their behaviors, thoughts, and feelings interact. For example, one young adult client came to the session saying that she had a very good week, except that she had slept badly on one night. She expressed a great deal of concern about this one night because "it was completely inexplicable," and it added to her growing anxiety that she had lost control over her sleep. So we went through, step-by-step in a very detailed way, her activities, thoughts, and feelings that day and evening. She was at work from 8:00 A.M. through 6:30 P.M., and the day was stressful. At 7:00 P.M. she arrived home. She found that her housemates had asked a bunch of her friends over, and they were all sitting around the living room. The client really wanted some quiet time for herself, so she went downstairs to do her laundry. On her way she happened to notice that there were lots of messages on her phone. She felt stressed that she didn't have the opportunity to return the calls. At 10:30 P.M. all of her friends relocated to a café, and she went along too. At 11:50 P.M. she returned home and went straight to bed thinking, "I must get to sleep quickly so I can cope at work tomorrow." This close analysis gave us clear clues as to why the client had a poor night of sleep—not enough time to herself, overwhelmed with people and things to do, no time to wind down before getting into bed, and putting pressure on herself to fall asleep quickly. Working this out increased the control felt by the client and created an opportunity to reinforce the cognitive-behavioral model. In other words, the teaching point to draw out is that when we examine the cognitions, behaviors, and emotions experienced in a situation, these kinds of experiences make more sense and lessen the thoughts that many clients with sleep problems have of feeling out of control, which contributes to anxiety (which, of course, exacerbates the sleep problem). This process also points to the possibility of amending the treatment plan by including a focus on the strategies for managing stress at work (Optional Module 4) and for developing an individualized wind-down, including less exposure to the telephone or cellphone (Core Module, Part B).

Combining the Functional Analysis and the Assessment

With the functional analysis, daily sleep diary, and the PROMIS scales and other parts of the assessment completed, it is time to combine this knowledge in a way that provides a road map for administering the core and optional modules of TranS-C. The daily sleep diary for the 14-year-old female featured in Box 3.1 is presented in Figure 3.1. (For this case, we used a modified version of the sleep diary, to make it more appropriate for the teenage client to use.) Below the diary, the therapist has added the calculations needed to evaluate the six sleep health dimensions. With respect to these dimensions, the information given in the completed diary suggests the following:

- *Regularity.* A review of the bedtimes and wake times indicates considerable fluctuation from night to night. Ideally we would like to see minimal night-to-night fluctuation in both times.

- *Satisfaction with sleep.* For this client we modified the sleep diary, including removing the sleep quality question. However, we do have this client's score on the sleep quality question of the PROMIS Sleep Disturbance scale. On a scale from 1 "very poor" to 5 "very good," the client indicated that her sleep quality was 2. Ideally we would like to see ratings of 4 or 5 on this question.

- *Alertness during waking hours.* The client is napping most weekday afternoons for 15–90 minutes. Also, on the PROMIS Sleep-Related Impairment sale, the question about whether the client experienced daytime sleepiness was rated a 4 on a scale from 1 ("not at all") to 5 ("very much"). Together these data indicate that daytime alertness is quite a problem for this teenage client.

- *Timing of sleep.* Ideally the mid-sleep times (MSTs) would fall within the range of 2:00 A.M. to 4:00 A.M. for adults and perhaps earlier for teenagers who have a greater sleep need than adults, and who typically need to awaken early for school. As evident from this client's sleep diary, most of the MSTs are outside of this range. Also, when observing the timing of wake time it becomes clear that the client probably didn't make it to school on 2 days. This was confirmed by the client who said she was too tired to go to school.

- *Sleep efficiency.* SE is very low across the week, varying from 37 to 62%. SE is calculated by dividing TST by TIB and multiplying the result by 100. The TIB evident in the diary is striking, varying from around 7 hours up to 17 hours. The client confirmed that this pattern is typical for her and that she tends to stay in bed when she feels depressed.

- *Sleep duration.* Mean TST based on the sleep diary varies from around 3.5 hours per night up to 7.5 hours per night, falling far short of the recommended 8.5 to 9.25 hours per night for teens.

Combining this information together with the modifiable maintaining behaviors and cognitions evident from Box 3.1, the cross-cutting and core modules of TranS-C will be a good match to this client's needs and will be used as the basic building blocks for improving her sleep health. In terms of the optional modules, the information gathered indicates that the following modules need to be provided: Optional Module 1, because the client's SE is well below the target of 85%; Optional Module 2, as there is a need to reduce the total amount of time the client is in bed; and Optional Module 3, given the evidence for delayed sleep onset times. In addition, her concern about her boyfriend and school indicates that Optional Module 4, which is focused on reducing sleep-related vigilance, should be also be provided. Note that the DSISD did not raise concerns about comorbid sleep disorders, such as sleep apnea. Remember that while the ordering of the various TranS-C modules in

My Sleep Diary

	Example Monday 8/7	Thursday 10/19	Friday 10/20	Saturday 10/21	Sunday 10/22	Monday 10/23	Tuesday 10/24	Wednesday 10/25
The morning I filled out the diary for last night was . . .								
1. What time did you get into bed last night?	11:00 A.M. / (P.M.)	12:00 (A.M.) / P.M.	10:00 A.M. / (P.M.)	11:30 A.M. / (P.M.)	11:00 A.M. / (P.M.)	11:00 A.M. / (P.M.)	10:30 A.M. / (P.M.)	11:00 A.M. / (P.M.)
2. What time did you try to go to sleep?	11:30 A.M. / (P.M.)	12:45 (A.M.) / P.M.	1:00 (A.M.) / P.M.	2:00 (A.M.) / P.M.	2:00 (A.M.) / P.M.	1:30 (A.M.) / P.M.	12:00 (A.M.) / P.M.	12:30 (A.M.) / P.M.
3. How long did it take you to fall asleep?	30 min	100 min	60 min	30 min	60 min	43 min	45 min	3½ hours
4. How many times did you wake up, not counting your final awakening?	1	0	0	0	0	1	0	0
5. For how long did each awakening last?	10 min	N/A	N/A	N/A	N/A	10 min	N/A	N/A
6. What time was your final awakening?	6:50 (A.M.) / P.M.	6:50 (A.M.) / P.M.	7:00 (A.M.) / P.M.	10:00 (A.M.) / P.M.	9:00 (A.M.) / P.M.	6:50 (A.M.) / P.M.	7:00 (A.M.) / P.M.	7:30 (A.M.) / P.M.
7. What time did you get out of bed for the day?	7:10 (A.M.) / P.M.	7:10 (A.M.) / P.M.	12:00 A.M. / (P.M.)	1:00 A.M. / (P.M.)	12:30 A.M. / (P.M.)	7:30 (A.M.) / P.M.	3:30 A.M. / (P.M.)	7:30 (A.M.) / P.M.

(continued)

FIGURE 3.1. Example of a completed sleep diary for a 14-year-old female.

8. Think back to yesterday, how many times did you nap or doze?	0	1	0	0	1	0	1
9. What time/s did you nap or doze?	N/A A.M. / P.M.	3:30 A.M. / (P.M.)	N/A A.M. / P.M.	N/A A.M. / P.M.	3:00 A.M. / (P.M.)	N/A A.M. / P.M.	3:30 A.M. / (P.M.)
10. In total, how long did you nap or doze?	N/A	15 min	N/A	N/A	90 min	N/A	60 min

TO BE COMPLETED BY CLINICIAN

Time in Bed (TIB)	7 hrs 10 min	14 hrs 00 min	13 hrs 30 min	13 hr 30 min	8 hrs 30 min	17 hrs 00 min	8 hrs 30 min
Total Sleep Time (TST)	4 hrs 25 min	5 hrs 00 min	7 hrs 30 min	6 hrs 00 min	4 hrs 27 min	6 hrs 15 min	3 hrs 30 min
Sleep Efficiency (SE)	62%	36%	56%	44%	52%	37%	41%
Midsleep Time (MST)	3:35 A.M.	5:00 A.M.	6:15 A.M.	5:45 A.M.	3:15 A.M.	7:00 A.M.	3:15 A.M.

Weekly Average Values
TIB: 11 hrs 44 min
TST: 5 hrs 18 min
SE: 46.9%
MST: 4:52 A.M.

FIGURE 3.1. (continued)

61

Box 1.2 is useful for many clients, it is important to be sensitive to differences between patients as to which processes are most strongly contributing to their distress, so that those processes can be addressed at an earlier stage of treatment. Because we did not have any indication that a reordering of the modules is warranted with this client, we proceeded with the cross-cutting modules first.

Additional Considerations

During this early phase of treatment there are several other issues that commonly arise.

Client Expectations

Many small changes can eventually amount to a profound, qualitative change. Some clients and therapists are looking for the *one* factor they can *fix* that will magically resolve the sleep problem. This is rarely realistic. The focus of TranS-C is on making multiple small adjustments that add up to a major change in a client's sleep experience. We explain this to clients by using a cookie recipe metaphor: Just as it takes many ingredients to make a good cookie, it similarly takes many tweaks to make a good sleeper.

For one adolescent client, the possible contributors to his sleep problem that became apparent from the case formulation were the following:

- Mom or Dad would check on him throughout the night. This attention made him vigilant, which made it difficult to drop off to sleep.
- The client said he tried to "clear thoughts from his mind." This is a form of thought suppression that typically leads to further rebound in the thoughts.
- The client monitored the clock, which increased his anxiety, arousal, and frustration.
- The client expected to sleep poorly, and he estimated that he had a low chance of falling asleep. These expectations also contributed to anxiety and arousal.
- The client extended *a lot* of effort to sleep well (e.g., he would arrange nine pillows around his body, which had to be arranged in a specific way; he would lie in bed and "work hard" to push his body into the sleep state).

In this case reversing each of these processes involved many small adjustments to the client's behavior and his beliefs about sleep.

Time Frame for Change

Take care to set realistic expectations for the time frame over which sleep improvements will be experienced. For example, if a client reduces caffeine use for 1 day, he or she is unlikely to see a sleep difference immediately. Similarly, if a client starts a morning habit of bright light exposure (e.g., opening the blinds to look out), it is unlikely to see immediate results. In general, we suggest explaining to clients that multiple adjustments typically need to be made, and that their impact will generally emerge over a 2- to 3-week period. Point out that the experience is similar to the fatigue from jet leg, in which the body needs to adjust to a new time zone or to acclimating to daylight saving time. The most time each day that our brains can adjust to is 1 hour. So it really does take a couple of weeks to adjust to a new schedule and routine.

"This Is All Biological"

The client may want to talk about whether his or her sleep problem is a biological or a psychological problem. This commonly occurs when clients believe the problem is biological and are confused as to why they are participating in a psychosocial treatment. For these clients, we explain that the biological, psychological, and social domains are intimately intertwined in the realm of sleep, and that a change in one domain will result in a change to another. For example, moving into dim light conditions around bedtime (a behavior) will trigger a biological change (the release of melatonin by the pineal gland).

"I've Tried That"

Some clients may have already tried components of TranS-C that they have found on the Internet, with little success, and are reluctant to try the same strategy again. In these cases we begin by assessing exactly what was tried and over what time frame. It is not uncommon to find that the strategy was incompletely implemented or was not tried for long enough. Multiple adjustments are typically needed for improving sleep, so it is not uncommon to find that the strategy was implemented incompletely or not long enough. Often the Internet presentation of the treatment modules is lacking in the rationale for the recommendations. Hence, grounding the recommendations in the sleep and circadian science (Cross-Cutting Module 2) can be very helpful.

Psychosis: Voices and Visions That Interfere with Sleep

There is evidence for a bidirectional causal relationship between sleep disturbance and psychotic experiences, whereby sleep disturbance increases the experience of psychotic symptoms and psychotic symptoms increase sleep dis-turbance (Freeman et al., 2010; Freeman, Pugh, Vorontsova, & Southgate, 2009; Freeman et al., 2012). For example, Waite et al. (2015) document that a client described how "the voices wrecked my sleep" and that distressing voices prevented sleep onset: "I am trying to sleep and they [the voices] distract me and they keep me awake."

People who hear voices (auditory hallucinations) or see visions (visual hal-lucinations) often report that the voices and visions are worse at night when there are no distractions. We begin by doing a thorough assessment of what the voices say and the type of visions experienced. We ask about the frequency of these occurrences (retrospective estimate) and add a row to the sleep diary noting the nights over the coming week when voices and visions are experi-enced (prospective data). Obtaining both the retrospective and prospective data is very helpful for establishing the frequency of these experiences. We also ask about the duration and the extent of the associated distress, along with the strategies (if any) the client has tried. Then we present the material in Optional Module 4, concentrating on the menu of options for managing unwanted thoughts, as well as the intervention for thought suppression. It can also be helpful to draw a distinction between what is real and what is not real. For example, with one client we developed this mantra: "The bed *is real*, I am safe—that *is real*, the voices/visions *are not real*."

In addition, feel free to be creative in experimenting with different tech-niques. For example, sometimes listening to a calming voice on the radio can help distract the client from the voices or visions. Suggest that the client try to use a radio that can automatically turn off after a period of time so it doesn't interfere with sleep later in the night. Getting up to go to another room also can be a helpful distraction from the voices/visions.

If Unsure, Collect Data

If a client reports bad dreams, ask him or her to start recording dreams in the sleep diary, and add a new row to the diary to facilitate this. If a client reports that her menstrual cycle is the cause of her sleep problems, ask her to keep a diary of her menstrual cycle alongside her sleep diary. If a client reports that his sleep problem is caused by back pain, add rows to the sleep diary to record pain ratings during the night and on waking each day. Also, ask about and write down the client's specific predictions before the data collection starts. For example, does the client believe he or she has bad dreams every night of the week? Does the client believe her sleep worsens the entire week prior to the beginning of her period, or is it just 2 days before? Each week examine the data together to determine whether it is consistent or inconsistent with the predictions. These data are always informative. Sometimes we discover that the dreams almost never occur and that the menstrual cycle has no bearing on the quality of sleep (this happens surprisingly often!). At other times the predictions are confirmed, and the data then direct us to spend time addressing this variable in treatment.

Cross-Cutting Module 2: Sleep and Circadian Education

This module has three goals: (1) to share knowledge about sleep and circadian rhythms, which continues the process of providing the rationale for TranS-C; (2) to impart a sense of curiosity about the wonders of sleep, which can help promote motivation to improve sleep; and (3) to start to craft the scientific rationale for the change that will promote sleep health.

We have developed a handout on the basics of sleep for adults in Appendix 4 and a developmentally appropriate handout for adolescents in Appendix 5. To promote engagement and a sense of curiosity about sleep, consider supplementing these handouts by selecting from the resources in Appendix 2 (other media relevant to specific interests/passions the client may have). While working through the handouts, pause regularly to encourage the client to ask questions and to determine which aspects of the material apply to the client's life.

There are several key "take-home" messages from this module:

- We often live our lives at such a fast pace that we risk losing touch with a fundamental, if neglected, fact: that our bodies and the physical world around us are governed by 24-hour rhythms. We may even try to medicate our rhythms—we drink caffeine or take some other kind of "upper" in the day, and we drink alcohol or take another kind of "downer" at night. This education module presents the rationale for recognizing, respecting, and regularizing body rhythms, particularly bedtimes and wake times. Good, basic knowledge about sleep and circadian rhythms helps clients to understand why their current sleep-related behaviors may not work well and why we are making specific recommendations.

- A basic introduction on the structure of sleep (sleep architecture) helps clients realize how important sleep is for many basic life functions, thereby increasing motivation to improve their sleep. Sleep consists of two major types: non-REM and REM, each with its own characteristic features and functions. Upon falling asleep we rapidly descend to the deepest stage of sleep, referred to as non-REM Stage N3. Stage N3 is important for the secretion of growth hormone, cellular repair, and immune system functioning; for helping us to retain long-term information and memories; and for balancing out the hormones that regulate our appetite and weight. We then ascend briefly into Stage N2 sleep, a lighter stage that helps to build and maintain muscle memory, like that needed for playing sports or other physical activities, prepares the brain for the next day's learning, and helps us integrate *new* information into *existing* memories. Stage N2 transitions into REM sleep, a relatively light stage of sleep during which most dreaming occurs. REM sleep is important for memory consolidation, emotional processing, and creativity. A typical night of sleep involves regular cycles of non-REM and REM sleep, which occur every 90–110 minutes. A number of brief awakenings with rapid return to sleep are also a feature of normal sleep architecture. Among adults there will be approximately four 90–110 minute cycles across the night, with REM occupying about 25% of the total in adults. However, sleep architecture varies across the age range, with infants having more REM and older adults having less non-REM Stage N3.

- The total amount of sleep also varies across the age range, with older adults needing less sleep—ideally about 7 hours per night. It is important to reassure clients that awakenings in the night are common and normal, and if we wake up midway through a sleep stage, when we resume sleeping we go back to the stage of sleep our body most needs.

- Sleep is controlled by two physiological processes: the homeostatic process and the circadian process. The homeostatic process can be described as the sleep "drive" or sleep "pressure" that accumulates with every moment we spend awake. This pressure to go to sleep increases more and more the longer we are awake, then drops back down to zero as we sleep at night. When we nap during the day, we discharge this pressure to sleep. So we have to be very careful about napping, and clients should be asked how often and for how long they nap each day. The circadian process refers to the rhythm in our bodies that follows a roughly 24-hour cycle. A circadian rhythm that is tightly synchronized to the daily light–dark cycle and to regular daily routines helps us to sleep better at night and stay awake during the day. Every day, we resynchronize with the help of cues such as regular breakfast and dinner times, a regular time for movement and exercise, a regular time for socializing, and for exposure to light—which is the most powerful of all the time cues.

- Light has a powerful influence on circadian rhythms via its action on a brain area known as the suprachiasmatic nucleus or SCN. The SCN is the body's master clock that serves to synchronize and time the rhythms of our physical, mental, and cognitive functions. As a particular example, the SCN controls the production of melatonin, a hormone that promotes sleepiness. Thus, a regular light–dark cycle helps the SCN to relay a strong 24-hour signal to the full range of body and brain rhythms, including the sleep–wake rhythm.

- Melatonin, a hormone regulated by the SCN and released by the pineal gland, can be thought of as a hormone of darkness that promotes sleep at night. Melatonin secretion by the pineal gland has a strong circadian pattern, being released only at night; however, its secretion is also very sensitive to environmental light and is released only if the environment is dark. In fact, light at night will suppress melatonin secretion, which may contribute to poor sleep. If we choose to be awake past a reasonable time and bathe ourselves in light, melatonin cannot kick in to help us fall asleep. We use this information to ask the client about light exposure, such as turning on a bright bathroom light when visiting the restroom during the night or using technology in bed or during the night. Helpful questions include: "What kinds of lights are you exposed to in the hours before bedtime?" and "What time do you switch off the lights at night?"

- Finally, we present the little known fact that the SCN in the human brain performs a role similar to that of an orchestra conductor: It has the challenge of keeping tens of thousands of different clocks in the body synchronized! Every cell and organ in the body has its own clock. It's a major challenge—critical to our health and well-being—to keep this orchestra of clocks synchronized. The best way to promote a tuneful orchestra in which all the clocks are "in time" is to wake up and go to bed around the same time each night. When we have very irregular sleep–wake schedules, we are living in a chronically jet-lagged state. For example, a 3-hour night-to-night difference in sleep during 1 week is like flying from New York to San Francisco on a weekly basis. We explore whether or not the client has experienced jet lag and what it was like. If the client has not, we share our own experience. For example, when we fly to New York from San Francisco, it's not possible to fall asleep at our normal San Francisco bedtime (10:00 P.M.) in New York, as the time would be 7:00 P.M. in San Francisco. The circadian system cannot make such a big leap in one day. Similarly, it's really hard to wake up at 7:00 A.M. for an 8:00 A.M. meeting in New York because the time would be 4:00 A.M. in San Francisco. Again, the circadian system cannot make such a large leap. The take-home message is that if we regularize our bedtimes and wake times for each week we don't need to deal with chronic jet lag.

- Two additional topics are addressed for adolescents. First, because the brain and body are still rapidly developing, adolescents need 8½ to 9¼ hours of sleep per night. Second, we discuss the possible reasons for teens use of technology at night: texting and social media are rewarding and fun; technology use constitutes time away from parents/guardians; and it addresses the social concerns some teens feel such as FOMO (fear of missing out), fear of being alone, and fear of bullying or exclusion if disconnected.

Promote Active Engagement When Sharing Handouts

We suggest the therapist ask the client, "Would you like me to read, or do you want to read, or should we share the reading?" Try to share reading the handouts, as sharing will promote his or her active involvement. Pause regularly to give your own examples, elicit examples from the client, and discuss the key points. For example, to illustrate the homeostatic and circadian sleep drives, ask if the client ever stayed up all night and remembers how he or she felt the next day. Some therapists throw out fun "quick-quiz" questions to make the psychoeducation more of a game. This works very well, particularly with teenagers. For example: "In your own words what does melatonin do?"

Cross-Cutting Module 3: Behavior Change and Motivation

> We must make automatic and habitual, as early as possible, as many useful actions as we can. . . . The more details of our daily life we can hand over to the effortless custody of automatism, the higher mental powers of mind will be set free for their own proper work.
> —WILLIAM JAMES (1842–1910)

Poor adherence to treatment recommendations is a major and complex problem in almost all client populations, medical specialties, and settings. Nonadherence is associated with poor clinical outcomes. Also, some clients come to treatment as "prisoners" because their parent, doctor, or case manager insists that they attend. Our challenge is to work creatively to find the motivational levers that turn "prisoners" into "customers." Another commonly encountered problem for clients is making the transition from learning about the reasons for their sleep problems to changing their behaviors. Also, there is a subgroup of clients, particularly adolescents, who have difficulty adapting to a schedule that enables them to wake up in time for school or work feeling refreshed but who are not particularly troubled by their late schedule or lack of sleep. Unless we are able to find intrinsic motivators for these clients, they are very unlikely to respond to treatment. Examples of such motivators include becoming a better athlete, feeling happier and less moody, performing better at school or work, and getting along better with peers and family members. Resources that build on these and other motivational levers are available in Appendix 2. TranS-C draws on the science of behavior change and habit formation to optimize its delivery, particularly with clients who are experiencing low or mixed motivation, and to ensure lasting change.

For each segment of treatment we spend time discussing how the material is relevant to the client's life by asking at regular intervals, "Which of these sleep domains are relevant to you?" or "Based on the content, would you like to set some goals for this coming week? If so, what should those goals be, and what are the obstacles to achieving these goals." If the client doesn't come up with any ideas or is resistant, the therapist can choose between two options:

1. Revisiting the topic at a later date if you hypothesize that the topic is highly relevant to the client. Sometimes the client is more open the second time around.
2. Making one or more suggestions about an experiment or a goal and see whether the client is interested (if not, return to Option 1). For this option, it is very important to explain the rationale for the suggestion you are making.

This treatment module also addresses fostering new habits to replace unhelpful habits. A common example is the use of technology in bed, which continues to be very widespread (90% of people in one survey; Gradisar et al., 2013), despite strong arguments against its use.

We propose a number of steps to achieving lasting behavior change and habit formation.

Normalize That Change Is Difficult

This is a first step in the process of behavior change. Forming new habits is not easy. For example, a very insightful 48-year-old client diagnosed with schizophrenia observed how hard it is for him to get out of his chair while watching television each morning. He noted that he would rather go to the gym or for a walk, but he found it impossible to get himself out of the chair. The therapist said, "I certainly empathize with you. I don't find it easy to switch the television off; it's so comfortable and engaging. I think a lot of people have this experience."

It's also important to note that although most of us understand that we should adopt healthy behaviors, we don't actually do so. This gap between understanding and doing is captured beautifully in a paper by Casagrande, Wang, Anderson, and Gary (2007). These authors document that, although we all know that a diet high in fruits and vegetables is associated with decreased risk of cardiovascular disease, cancer, and diabetes, only 11% of people meet the guidelines of eating two servings of fruit and three servings of vegetables recommended per day. Thus, an essential aspect of TranS-C is normalizing the almost universal difficulty of forming new healthy habits.

Develop a Compelling Rationale for Change

Collaborate with the client to explore why making a change is important. The rationale needs to be linked to the client's experience, personal goals, and their sleep habits. We borrow tools from MI (Miller & Rollnick, 2013) for this purpose. MI has been used with a broad range of client groups, including those with substance use problems, eating disorders, physical health problems, obesity, parent-child interaction problems, and oral health problems. Rubak, Sandbæk, Lauritzen, and Christensen (2005) conducted a review and meta-analysis of 72 randomized controlled trials of MI and found that MI had a significant and clinically relevant effect in three out of four studies, with a similar effect on physiological and psychological problems.

The core values within the MI approach are non-judgment, empathy, and collaboration. MI is done *for* and *with* clients; it is not done *to* them. When a client's ambivalence tips toward change, discussion can begin about when and how to change.

MI assumes that ambivalence about change is normal and that clients will already have arguments for and against change in their heads. While it might be a natural inclination to argue for change, this is a mistake. Arguing for change evokes the other side of the client's ambivalence, against change. Instead of arguing for or giving advice about change, we listen to the client and ask open-ended questions designed to elicit his or her own reasons for changing, called "change talk." For example:

> "Why would you want to make this change?"
> "How might you go about it in order to succeed?"
> "What are the three best reasons for you to do it?"
> "How important is it for you to make this change and why?"
> "So what do you think you'll do?" (Miller & Rollnick, 2013, p. 11)

Another important MI tool is developing with the client a list of the pros and cons of making a change, and of not making a change. Try to acquire the habit of fluidly interweaving MI by conducting a review of the cons and then the pros of trying the homework and of not trying the homework each week. We often find it helpful to review the pros after we promote "change talk." We review the cons first to reveal the obstacles to change that can then be discussed and resolved.

Collaborate on How, When, and Where the New Behavior Will Be Implemented

Brainstorm the options together with the client. Consider using and teaching the client to use one or both of the following evidence-based visualization strategies developed by cognitive psychologists to aid implementation. These approaches are useful for reviewing and summarizing the implementation plan (Harvey et al., 2014).

Implementation intentions are simple, quick techniques that take advantage of mental imagery in deciding how to implement one's goals. They general format of this technique involves identifying a goal, then asking participants to say out loud or to themselves their commitment to pursuing their goal. We recommend using a form like: "If/when I encounter this situation _____, I intend to _____ at this time _____ in this _____ place." The client is then asked to write down his or her commitment, to visualize the situation and response as vividly as possible, and then to repeat the process a few times. The results of studies on implementation intentions are quite staggering. In a meta-analysis of published findings from 94 tests, implementation intentions had a positive effect of medium-to-large magnitude on goal attainment (Gollwitzer & Sheeran, 2006). It is thought that the mental representation established by forming an implementation intention signified that the plan is "highly activated and thus more easily accessible" (Gollwitzer, 1999, p. 495).

Mental contrasting is a technique that involves conjoint mental elaboration of the desired future and the present reality, thereby making both present and future simultaneously accessible and creating strong associations between them (Oettingen et al., 2009). The general format involves encouraging the client to fantasize about a positive future—for example: "What is it that would make it so good for you personally to seize your goal? Let's spend a few minutes imagining your response as vividly as possible. Let yourself indulge in fantasizing about this positive outcome without considering obstacles in the present reality." Then the contrast is introduced—for example: "What is the most critical obstacle that stands in the way of you seizing your goal? Let's spend a few minutes imagining the most critical obstacle as vividly as possible." Again, the effects on future behavior are staggering. It is thought that the simultaneous activation of the desired future and present reality emphasizes the necessity for action. When expectations of success are high, mental contrasting is thought to energize individuals to take action, thereby strengthening their goal commitment.

Implementation intentions and mental contrasting techniques have been combined in a study of adolescents preparing to take an exam. The students who participated in the combined use of implementation intentions and mental contrasting completed 60 more study questions (Duckworth, Grant, Loew,

Oettingen, & Gollwitzer, 2011). Appendix 6 includes the worksheet that helps guide clients through the combined use of these two strategies.

Uncover and Understand the Real and Perceived Barriers to Behavior Change

Some examples of these barriers to change that should be explored with clients include an uncomfortable bed, a bedroom that is noisy or not dark enough, a roommate who insists on the light being on during the night, noisy neighbors, and so forth.

Repetition and Practice Are Essential to Habit Formation

This is captured in a famous aphorism attributed to Aristotle: "We are what we repeatedly do. Excellence, then, is not an act, but a habit." By practicing new behaviors over and over, they become automatic tendencies that are not mediated by active mental representations of goals. In other words, once habits are formed, they are enacted even in the absence of conscious intent and are not disrupted by lapses of attention, changes in motivation, or stress. Once the association is formed, perceiving the appropriate cue will automatically retrieve the response from memory and trigger an impulse to initiate it (Galla & Duckworth, 2015). For example, the wind-down component of TranS-C should be practiced so often that when clients perceive the time to be 1 hour before bedtime, they automatically start their wind-down (e.g., turning off the computer or TV, feeding the pets, washing or showering, etc.)

Build Bundles of Behaviors into the Routine

For example, rather than working on morning bright light exposure in isolation, TranS-C emphasizes establishing a morning routine consisting of multiple components that are practiced together as a bundle. An example is a group of strategies called the "RISE-UP" routine covered in Core Module 1 (see Chapter 4). The specific bundle of strategies varies from person to person. One bundle of strategies could be to get out of bed as soon as the alarm goes off, to open the curtains or blinds to let daylight in, to make the bed so it's harder to get back in, to head straight for the shower, to dress, and then go straight to the kitchen, letting the daylight in, and to enjoy coffee and breakfast.

Monitor Progress toward Goals

Brainstorm together with the client how he or she can record trying the new behavior (e.g., adding a row to the daily sleep diary). Recording new behaviors is key because we know that monitoring is associated with improvement in goal attainment (Harkin et al., 2016). Any progress should be recognized and reinforced. Inquire as to how the client managed to achieve the goal, even in the smallest way. Then complete a functional analysis to begin to understand why the client was unable to engage with the plan on other nights and find a way for the client to do so more fully over the coming week.

Promote the Client Remembering the Plan

Write down a "sleep prescription" for the client and ask, "What would help you remember to do this?"

Conduct a Functional Analysis If There Is No Change

If a client continues to find it difficult to change a problem behavior, review a recent episode in detail. Ask about the context and the client's thoughts, feelings, and behaviors. This practice very often reveals a set of targets for further exploration or intervention.

Other Tips for Building Motivation

Supplement the agenda with humorous or enjoyable add-ons, such as videos or articles based on the client's interests (see Appendices 1 and 2 for examples).

For some clients, the bed itself has become aversive. Explore why. Has negative conditioning taken place? Is being in bed boring? Does sleep feel like a waste of precious time? In other words, unpack and understand your client's experiences and perspectives.

For the many clients who have not voluntarily sought treatment (they have been referred by others) and are ambivalent about it, take on the challenge of turning these people into "customers." The strategies that follow have been helpful in these cases.

• Spend more time in Session 1 on sleep and circadian education (Cross-Cutting Module 2). Because the topic of sleep is inherently interesting to many people, educating clients about the sleep process can be an effective way of generating enthusiasm. For these clients we often leave goal setting for a later session. We time the goal setting for when the client becomes ready for action. Otherwise it can be difficult to get the client's buy-in on the goals.

• It is very important for clients to leave Session 1 feeling that the time they have spent has been used well and having a sense of hope that the treatment will offer enough rewards to make it worthwhile to return for Session 2. In our experience, spending at least some time on the sleep and circadian education (Cross-Cutting Module 2) serves this purpose.

- We are all different in terms of what motivates us. Keep an ear out for the client's "motivation levers," which are the things that fire that person up. Motivational levers emerge as we get to know the client and as the treatment unfolds and the conversation develops. For some of the adolescents we have worked with, common motivational levers are performing well at work or school and athletic performance. For some of our adult clients, being a good parent or partner or managing better at work are common motivational levers. Often multiple motivational levers can be uncovered. For one adult client, the reasons for improving his sleep included:

  ○ Improving sleep will reduce my bodily pain (there is much empirical evidence for a link between sleep and pain).
  ○ Improving sleep will increase my chance of getting a job.
  ○ Improving sleep will increase my chance of keeping a job.
  ○ Improving sleep will improve my overall health (evidence shows that when people are sleeping well they lose weight and their blood pressure and their immunity improve).

Once a motivational lever is uncovered, we recommend providing regular reminders of the connection between improved sleep and these motivators.

Cross-Cutting Module 4: Goal Setting

Goal setting provides a focus for treatment and for monitoring progress. It is also a source of useful information about the client's expectations about their sleep and provides an opportunity to correct unhelpful or unrealistic expectations.

During the completion of Cross-Cutting Models 1 and 2, the goals for treatment will have started to emerge. A discussion of goals could start with a question like: "Given all that we've discussed, what goals do you think we ought to work toward for your sleep?" Add your suggestions for worthwhile goals to the discussion.

Set goals for the night and goals for the day. The daytime goals are important since daytime impairment is an essential feature of sleep problems (American Academy of Sleep Medicine, 2005; American Psychiatric Association, 2013; Edinger, Bonnet, et al., 2004). While there is evidence that improving nighttime sleep improves daytime functioning (Harvey, Bélanger, et al., 2014; Kyle, Morgan, Spiegelhalder, & Espie, 2011), other research raises the possibility that the nighttime and daytime aspects of sleep problems may be functionally independent (Lichstein et al., 2001; Neitzert Semler & Harvey, 2005). Hence, TranS-C includes a module focusing on the daytime aspects of sleep problems.

Make sure that goals are realistic, specific, and measurable. As discussed earlier in this chapter, we often add questions to the daily sleep diary to track goals session by session.

- *Examples of realistic and specific nighttime goals:* Get into bed by 10:00 P.M., get to sleep by 10:20 P.M., and turn off the phone 1 hour before bed. (Do not use "sleep more," which is too vague.)
- *Examples of realistic and specific daytime goals:* Wake up at the same time on weekdays and weekends, get out of bed within 10 minutes of waking up, stop snoozing. (Do not use "feel better in the morning," which is too vague.)

Most people with sleep problems simply want to get "a good night of sleep." However, people attach different meanings to this concept. For some people, it means uninterrupted sleep. And, for others, it means deep sleep. It is important to unpack the meaning of these descriptions and correct unrealistic beliefs about what constitutes a good night's sleep. For example:

- For a client who wants "uninterrupted" sleep, we let them know that brief awakenings during the night are common and normal, particularly as we move through the age range.

- For a client who wants more "deep sleep," we explain that all humans get the deeper stages of sleep. We are hardwired for this, so it's not realistic to make getting "deeper sleep" a goal. Instead, therapists should use what they already know about the client to negotiate a revised goal that is realistic and measurable. For a client who has reported that worrying makes it difficult for her to get to sleep and stay asleep, you might say something like, "We find that the feeling of sleeping lightly is very common among folks who experience a lot of worries. Sometimes it's as if our worries keep happening during sleep. So I wonder what you would think about us setting a goal of reducing worrying before and during sleep. Might that be of interest to you?"

- For a client who wishes to fall asleep the moment his or head hits the pillow, educate him that sleep onset is more like dimming a light rather than turning off a light. It typically takes normal sleepers 20 or so minutes to fall to sleep once in bed. Each sleep–wake transition (getting to sleep at the beginning of the night and waking up in the morning) takes time.

• If a client's goal is to "feel better in the morning," it is important to point out (1) that ultimately the best way to feel better in the morning might be to rework the sleep–wake schedule to improve sleep along the six sleep health dimensions and (2) that due to sleep inertia—the transitional phase between sleep and wake—very few people are energetic immediately on waking. It is normal to feel groggy. This topic is covered in more detail in Chapter 5.

• If a client states a goal of getting less sleep or more sleep, consider saying something along the lines of "You also mentioned that you would like to get 6 or 7 hours of sleep a night (or 9 or 10 hours of sleep a night). The research on sleep suggests that most adults do best on 7–8 hours. Would you be interested in setting a goal of sleeping around 8 hours per night?"

These educational points prompt discussion about more realistic goals and begin the process of identifying and correcting unhelpful beliefs about sleep, which we cover in Chapter 5. A handout for recording separate daytime and nighttime goals nighttime is available as Appendix 7.

Link the client's sleep goals to his or her motivational levers. For example, one 15-year-old mentioned that he was excited to be applying for weekend jobs to save up for a car. However, every afternoon after school he napped for 90 minutes, which contributed to his maintaining very late night bedtimes. To help motivate this client to drop the naps, the therapist asked if the teen thought the boss would allow him to nap in the afternoon on a work day. That question motivated him to cut out after-school naps, which made it easier to set and earlier bedtime and achieve more sleep overall. Other motivational levers that can inspire youth to set bold goals for more sleep are the following: (1) the brain continues to develop up until 25 years of age, and sleep is critical for brain development; (2) sleep is important for body growth, muscle development, and sports; and (3) sleep is important for concentrating, learning, remembering, and doing well at school.

Therapy goals are typically set in Session 1 or 2 but they may need to be reevaluated and readjusted periodically as the intervention unfolds. Also, it is important to be clear that the initial goals are long range, meaning that the client is shooting to achieve them by the end of the treatment. Each week the client will take small steps toward these goals. For example, one teen started treatment with an average bedtime of 12:30 A.M. One of her long-range goals was to have a consistent 10:00 P.M. bedtime. She worked toward this goal over the course of treatment by shifting her bedtime 30 minutes earlier each week, allowing time for the circadian system to adjust. Trying for a bedtime of 10:00 P.M. the first week will likely result in the teen lying in bed awake and frustrated for 2½ hours.

An Exception to Setting a Specific Long-Range Goal

Usually we make sure that the goals set in the early sessions are specific. However, one exception is an eventual bedtime goal that is much earlier than the current bedtime, after considering the wake time for school or work and the client's sleep need. In this case, we have found that emphasizing the new bedtime goal of 10:00 P.M., for example, for someone who currently goes to bed at 1:00 A.M. may be demotivating and seem impossible for the client in Session 2. In these cases, consider whether it is appropriate to set a broader goal of "bringing bedtime forward" in Session 2. Get more specific as to what this means as progress is made and the new bedtime becomes more plausible.

CHAPTER 4

TranS-C Core Modules

The aim of this chapter is to introduce the four core modules of TranS-C. Core modules 1, 2, and 3 of TranS-C are powerful building blocks for healthy sleep. In our study with individuals diagnosed with bipolar disorder, progress in these three modules was often sufficient in improving sleep health (Kaplan & Harvey, 2013). Core Module 4, introduced in the last phase of treatment, aims to ensure that the gains made over the course of treatment are maintained after the treatment phase has drawn to a close.

Core Module 1: Establishing Regular Sleep–Wake Times

The sleep health framework that underpins TranS-C incorporates regularity in bedtimes and wake times as a core dimension (Buysse, 2014) given the evidence that irregularity is associated with poor school performance, mental illness, circadian rhythm disorders, negative health outcomes, and obesity (Bei et al., 2016).

Part A. Establishing Regular Sleep–Wake Times

One important goal is to set realistic and *regular* bedtimes and wake times. We suggest beginning by reviewing the daily sleep diary together with the client to ascertain whether irregular bedtimes and wake times are present and to ascertain the extent of day-to-day variability. Irregular bedtimes and wake times are usually salient features of most sleep diaries we review.

Figure 4.1 is the example of the daily sleep diary discussed in Chapter 2. From the answers to Question 5, it is evident that the night-to-night variability in the time this client tried to go to sleep was 5 hours (11:00 P.M. to 4:00 A.M.). From the answers to Question 9, we can see that the variability in wake times was 2½ hours (7:00 A.M. to 9:30 A.M.). Clearly the client who completed this diary is in need of this module! Moreover, note that the time this client got out of bed, in the answers to Question 10, varied from 7:00 A.M. to 11:00 A.M. This information is also relevant to this module, because it implies that the first meal of the day may have occurred anytime within a 4-hour window. Hence, we would regularize breakfast time as a way to support regular bedtimes and wake times. In a sense, this client's irregular sleep schedule is equivalent to flying through five time zones on a weekly basis! You might recall for the client the disruption you experience in your own sleep rhythms every time you travel over three time zones, and ask him or her to imagine doing this trip every week.

When the sleep diary indicates a need for regularizing sleep–wake times, as in Figure 4.1, the scientific rationale for this module should be explained. The key points are:

• The brain and body are highly rhythmic. Regular bedtimes and wake times support natural circadian (24-hour) rhythms. Irregular sleep–wake times dysregulate natural body rhythms and place the body in a state of chronic jet lag. In this state, obtaining the appropriate amount of sleep will not be possible.

• Regular wake-up times, in particular, are key to synchronizing our biological clock to the world outside us (i.e., entrainment) through regular exposure to light in the morning. This is the single most important timekeeper we have. Regular wake-up times also help us to regularize our other zeitgebers, such as the time we engage in physical activity, eating, and social activity.

• Every cell and organ of the human body has a biological clock. Regular sleep–wake times help keep this orchestra of biological clocks "in tune," which is important for health and well-being.

• Daytime or evening napping is typically an obstacle to establishing a regular bedtime, because napping discharges the homeostatic pressure to sleep.

• Aligning bedtimes and wake times become more attainable if we also work toward regularizing social rhythms (e.g., timing of meals, exercise, socializing, etc.).

• We will get our most satisfying sleep when we're in the habit of going to bed and waking up at regular times. This will ensure that the homeostatic pressure to sleep (or "sleep appetite") and the circadian pressure peak at the same time.

My Sleep Diary

Date	Example 1/9/17	7/26/17	7/27/17	7/28/17	7/29/17	7/30/17	7/31/17	8/1/17
Day	Monday	Wednesday	Thursday	Friday	Saturday	Sunday	Monday	Tuesday
For which night's sleep?	Sunday	Tuesday	Wednesday	Thursday	Friday	Saturday	Sunday	Monday
1. Please list the time and length of naps you took yesterday.	11:30–11:45 P.M. 3–5 P.M.	0	20 min 2 p.m.	0	0	20 min 1:00 p.m.	0	0
2a. How many drinks containing alcohol did you have yesterday?	2 drinks	0 drinks	0 drinks	0 drinks	0 drinks	0 drinks	0 drinks	0 drinks
2b. What time was your last alcoholic drink?	7:30 A.M. / (P.M.)	N/A A.M. / P.M.	N/A A.M. / P.M.	N/A A.M. / P.M.	N/A A.M. / P.M.	N/A A.M. / P.M.	N/A A.M. / P.M.	N/A A.M. / P.M.
3a. How many caffeinated drinks (coffee, tea, soda, energy drinks) did you have yesterday?	3 drinks	0 drinks	0 drinks	0 drinks	2 drinks	0 drinks	1 drinks	0 drinks

(continued)

FIGURE 4.1. Example of a completed sleep diary.

	Day 1	Day 2	Day 3	Day 4	Day 5	Day 6	Day 7	Day 8
3b. What time was your last caffeinated drink?	8:00 (A.M.) / P.M.	N/A A.M. / P.M.	N/A A.M. / P.M.	N/A A.M. / P.M.	N/A A.M. / P.M.	N/A A.M. / P.M.	N/A A.M. / P.M.	N/A A.M. / P.M.
4. What time did you get into bed last night?	12:45 (A.M.) / P.M.	1:30 (A.M.) / P.M.	11:45 A.M. / (P.M.)	11:30 A.M. / (P.M.)	11:00 A.M. / (P.M.)	11:00 A.M. / (P.M.)	4:00 (A.M.) / P.M.	10:30 A.M. / (P.M.)
5. What time did you try to go to sleep?	1:15 (A.M.) / P.M.	1:30 (A.M.) / P.M.	11:45 A.M. / (P.M.)	11:30 A.M. / (P.M.)	11:00 A.M. / (P.M.)	11:00 A.M. / (P.M.)	4:00 (A.M.) / P.M.	11:00 A.M. / (P.M.)
6. How long did it take you to fall asleep?	___ hr(s) 30 min(s)	___ hr(s) 30 min(s)	___ hr(s) 30 min(s)	___ hr(s) 30 min(s)	___ hr(s) 0 min(s)	___ hr(s) 20 min(s)	___ hr(s) 20 min(s)	___ hr(s) 30 min(s)
7. How many times did you wake up, not counting your final awakening?	2 times	2 times	2 times	1 times	0 times	2 times	0 times	2 times
8. For how long did each awakening last?	1st awakening ___ hr(s) 30 min(s) 2nd awakening 1 hr(s) 30 min(s) 3rd awakening ___ hr(s) ___ min(s)	1st awakening ___ hr(s) 30 min(s) 2nd awakening ___ hr(s) 30 min(s) 3rd awakening ___ hr(s) ___ min(s)	1st awakening 3 hr(s) ___ min(s) 2nd awakening 1 hr(s) ___ min(s) 3rd awakening ___ hr(s) ___ min(s)	1st awakening 3 hr(s) ___ min(s) 2nd awakening ___ hr(s) ___ min(s) 3rd awakening ___ hr(s) ___ min(s)	1st awakening ___ hr(s) ___ min(s) 2nd awakening ___ hr(s) ___ min(s) 3rd awakening ___ hr(s) ___ min(s)	1st awakening ___ hr(s) 30 min(s) 2nd awakening ___ hr(s) 30 min(s) 3rd awakening ___ hr(s) ___ min(s)	1st awakening ___ hr(s) ___ min(s) 2nd awakening ___ hr(s) ___ min(s) 3rd awakening ___ hr(s) ___ min(s)	1st awakening ___ hr(s) 20 min(s) 2nd awakening ___ hr(s) 20 min(s) 3rd awakening ___ hr(s) ___ min(s)

(continued)

FIGURE 4.1. *(continued)*

81

9. What time was your final awakening?	7:45 (A.M.)/P.M.	9:30 (A.M.)/P.M.	8:00 (A.M.)/P.M.	7:00 (A.M.)/P.M.	8:00 (A.M.)/P.M.	8:00 (A.M.)/P.M.	7:30 (A.M.)/P.M.	7:40 (A.M.)/P.M.
10. What time did you get out of bed for the day?	7:45 (A.M.)/P.M.	9:30 (A.M.)/P.M.	11:00 (A.M.)/P.M.	7:00 (A.M.)/P.M.	8:30 (A.M.)/P.M.	9:00 (A.M.)/P.M.	7:30 (A.M.)/P.M.	8:00 (A.M.)/P.M.
11. How would you rate the quality of your sleep last night?	1 (poor)	5	2	3	7	4	5	4

1   2   3   4   5   6   7
Poor Sleep Quality   Excellent Sleep Quality

TO BE COMPLETED BY CLINICIAN

Time in Bed (TIB)	8 hrs 00 min	11 hrs 15 min	7 hrs 30 min	9 hrs 30 min	10 hrs 00 min	3 hrs 30 min	9 hrs 30 min	
Total Sleep Time (TST)	6 hrs 30 min	3 hrs 45 min	4 hrs 00 min	9 hrs 00 min	7 hrs 40 min	3 hrs 10 min	7 hrs 30 min	
Sleep Efficiency (SE)	81%	33%	53%	95%	77%	90%	79%	
Midsleep Time (MST)	5:30 A.M.	5:24 A.M.	3:15 A.M.	3:45 A.M.	4:00 A.M.	5:45 A.M.	3:15 A.M.	

Weekly Average Values
TIB: 8 hrs 28 min
TST: 5 hrs 56 min
SE: 72.7%
MST: 4:24 A.M.

FIGURE 4.1. (continued)

82

Emphasize to the client that the process of aligning bedtimes and wake times typically takes several weeks. After examining the sleep diary with the client, set a long-range goal for aligning sleep–wake times. These are the goals the client is aiming for by the *end* of treatment. For the client who produced the sleep diary in Figure 4.1, a long-range goal of setting a bedtime at midnight and a wake time of 8:30 A.M. was proposed. It is important to be sensitive to the fact that some clients are best helped by setting a specific time (i.e., 8:30 A.M.), whereas other clients do better if a range is given (i.e., 8:00 A.M. to 9:00 A.M.). The specific times are decided after a discussion with the client based on his or her preferences (e.g., the time a favorite TV news program ends) and needs (e.g., the time the client has to be up for work). This decision provides a sleep window of 8½ hours in bed and acknowledges that it can take 15–20 minutes to fall to sleep once the light is turned off. It also takes into account that people tend to wake up in the night once or twice, perhaps to use the bathroom or to turn over. Then they take a few minutes to get back to sleep. Overall, if the client gets 8 hours of sleep in this 8½-hour window, sleep efficiency would be 94%, which is very good (recall that we aim for sleep efficiency for adults that is greater than 85% and 80% for older adults). We also set short-term or week-by-week goals, which are small steps in making progress toward the long-term goal. For example, for the client who produced the daily sleep diary in Figure 4.1, a short-term goal for the coming week was to try to establish bedtimes within 2 hours of the new goal and wake times within 1 hour of the new goal.

After the initial session of this module is finished, devote time in each subsequent session to reviewing the most recent daily sleep diary to monitor progression toward the bedtime and wake-time goals. Each week we determine how many nights the client managed to get into bed and wake up at the target time. Remember to recognize and verbally reinforce the efforts made by the client, even if he or she only managed to get into bed at the target time for just 1 night. For the nights the goal was achieved ask, "How were you able to achieve the goal on that night? What was different about it?" Then be curious about why the client didn't manage the target bedtime on the other nights. With this information in hand, we co-create a plan for the coming week to further improve regularizing the bedtime.

Commonly Encountered Problems

THE CLIENT FORGETS THE SLEEP DIARY

One commonly encountered problem is that clients arrive at the session without their sleep diary. They either left the diary at home or forgot to complete it. If this occurs, we suggest two approaches for obtaining an estimate of the amount of sleep for the prior week. We complete the sleep diary in the session for just the prior night and then assess the extent to which the amount of sleep obtained in the previous night was typical of the amount of sleep obtained throughout the week. An alternative approach is to ask for a weekly average and the range—for example: "What time did you typically go to bed? What was an early night? And what was a late night?"

We stress the importance of reminding the client to bring in the sleep diary to every session. Consider using text messaging and email to help the client remember. As the core building block of all sessions, the sleep diary documents crucial information about the client's implementation of and progress in the core and optional modules. Remember to brainstorm the obstacles the client faces in keeping the sleep diary and work toward a creative solution to remove the obstacles.

NIGHT EATING

Waking up during the night to eat should be discouraged in most circumstances. Metabolism is at a low ebb during the night, and the body is not expecting nor needing food. If a client develops a habit of waking up and eating, he/she will often start waking up about the same time each night feeling hungry. Recent evidence shows that calories consumed at night are more likely to lead to weight gain than the same calories consumed during the day.

SCHEDULING DIFFICULTIES

We have encountered many different types of scheduling difficulties related to sleep. For example, one teen spent half the week at her mother's house, where the bedtime was 11:00 P.M. The other half of the week was spent at her father's house, where the bedtime was 9:00 P.M. In this case we negotiated with the parents to align their daughter's bedtimes. Another example involved a client, who met the diagnostic criteria for bipolar disorder, who spent 5 nights a week at her parents' home, where she shared a room with her 12-year-old sister. There was a strict 9:00 P.M. bedtime and 7:00 A.M. wake time for the benefit of the younger sister. The client spent the other 2 nights of the week at her boyfriend's house. The boyfriend finished work at 11:00 P.M. 5 nights a week. By the time her boyfriend picked her up and took her back to his house, she wouldn't get to bed before 1:00 A.M. To obtain sufficient sleep on these 2 nights, the client slept until 10:00 A.M. and also took a 3-to-4 hour nap the following day. In this case, the therapist began by being curious about what happened at the boyfriend's house between 11:00 P.M. and 1:00 A.M. and explored whether or not it was realistic to move the client's bedtime back by 60 minutes. The therapist also explored the setup of the parent's house and asked if there might be another place for the client to sleep. The therapist provided reminders of the scientific rationale behind why this irregular schedule upsets the body's natural rhythms. The client decided to share the information with her parents and her boyfriend. As a result of this process, the parents set up another bedroom for the client to use so that she could establish a more regular sleep–wake schedule.

Part B. Learning a Wind-Down Routine

We collaborate with the client to devise an individualized wind-down routine that supports the regular bedtimes. Clients typically need assistance in devising a wind-down of 30–60 minutes in which relaxing, sleep-enhancing activities are introduced in dim light conditions. This module also supports the circadian phase advance for clients who are evening types (or night owls).

The scientific rationale for this module has, in part, been covered in Chapter 3. We remind the client of these points. In particular, we reiterate that light has a powerful influence by means of the special brain area known as the suprachiasmatic nucleus (SCN). The SCN is the body's master clock that controls the production of melatonin, a hormone that promotes sleepiness, and it relays information from the eyes to the brain. When there is less light—like at night—the SCN tells the brain to make more melatonin, which makes us feel sleepy. In other words, dim light or darkness is an important part of the wind-down. We also explain that melatonin is released by the pineal gland, which is stimulated by darkness, and causes us to feel sleepy. Melatonin can be released only in the dark—not in the light! Of course, this is worth remembering because we can be awake way past a reasonable bedtime if the lights are kept bright, and our melatonin cannot kick in to help us fall asleep. We also emphasize that the bedroom should be cool, comfortable, and comforting, and that the wind-down period is not a time to think about, process, or worry about the day or about tomorrow.

A recap of these key points is included in Appendices 4, 5, and 8 that accompany this module. Recall from Chapter 3 that you can supplement your review of these handouts by selecting from the resources in Appendices 1 and 2. While working through the handouts, we recommend pausing regularly to encourage the client to ask questions and to determine the aspects of the material that apply to the client's experience.

The overall goal of this module is to establish a wind-down that the client looks forward to because it is nourishing and soothing. We use the My Wind-Down form (Appendix 9) to document the wind-down plan or to write out the plan for the wind-down on a blank sheet of paper. Trying out the plan is the homework for the coming week. Each subsequent week we devote time in the session to reviewing the number of nights the client has managed to start his or her wind-down at the target time and the extent to which the targeted bedtime was achieved. As noted earlier, remember to praise and verbally reinforce the client for any progress he or she has made, and then collaborate on creating a plan for the coming week that will enable the client to establish a good wind-down habit.

Clients with a circadian rhythm disorder advanced phase, who fall to sleep too early, will need some nighttime activities to help them to *stay awake longer*. The wind-down period for these clients will look very different. Working with clients who have this disorder will be addressed in Optional Module 3.

Commonly Encountered Problems

TECHNOLOGY USE

A central issue we face in this module is the use of technology (Internet, cell-phones, MP3 players) during the wind-down period before bed. Teens, in particular, use a huge range of technology (i.e., YouTube, Netflix, video games, texting, pornography, Instagram), and many of them find it hard to imagine a period of free time that doesn't involve the use of electronic devices. However, the use of these devices can interfere with sleep not only because they produce light, but also because they are very stimulating. With the help of the scientific rationale and a discussion of the pros and cons of technology use, enable the client to achieve the ideal scenario of voluntarily choosing an electronic curfew or "electronic vacation" of 30–60 minutes before bedtime. If the client agrees to this curfew, it is very important to spend time considering these questions: "What will it be like for you to turn off technology? Any thoughts on what you will do instead?" "You will be in darkness for a while before you drift off to sleep. What will that be like for you?" If this is a domain the client is concerned about, consider administering Optional Module 4, Reducing Sleep-Related Worry and Vigilance. The aim of this module is to assist the client in managing unwanted thoughts and in learning alternative positive thought management strategies (e.g., savoring, practicing gratitude). In other words, make sure a plan is in place for a viable and attractive alternative to technology use.

It is crucial to uncover and understand your client's experience and perspective on the use of technology around bedtime.

- Ask your client about a time she or he didn't have access to technology (e.g., camping). Explore what that experience was like; ask what the teen did instead.

- Many of our teens spend hours gaming each night. Be curious about the reasons for this. Ask the client questions to try and understand the motivation for gaming until late into the night. You may get more information if you ask, "Why do you think people your age spend hours gaming?" rather than "What do you like about gaming?"

● Try talking about short-term rewards (gaming) and longer-term rewards (being well rested, doing well at school, etc.).

● Consider asking the teen to take a video or picture of his or her bedroom. Having a picture might help you to understand where the lights and window coverings are situated in relation to the bed and how they might be moved to limit the amount of bright light the teen is exposed to at night.

● Suggest limiting the light emitted by devices by listening to an audiobook instead of watching a video or by turning down screen brightness.

● For teens who are text messaging their friends into the night, help your clients talk to their friends about switching off as a group.

● One teen watched 2 hours of pornography each night. His therapist helped him review his daily sleep diary and calculated his TST for this past week. Then they both discussed the teen's view on the pros and cons of increasing his total sleep time (from 5 hours per night), which they wrote down. The teen was then in a position to start thinking about how to improve his total sleep time. The therapist suggested doing experiments (e.g., 15 minutes of videos each night instead of 2 hours) to determine what might work best.

● Sometimes a client will not be willing to completely give up technology use. In these cases, we use a harm reduction approach in which we try to modify the client's use of technology in stages. This means exploring whether the client may be willing to move gradually in a healthier direction (e.g., reduce the light setting on an iPad, moving the TV further from his or her bed). To be effective, the technology intervention needs to be individualized. For example, for one teen we decided that 24 minutes of *Seinfeld* was better than a 1½-hour science fiction movie. Another teen found that reading was a problem—he couldn't put his book down for 1–2 hours. For him, one episode of *Seinfeld* was more helpful for falling asleep.

Bear in mind, however, that the scientific evaluation of the impact of technology use in youth is at an early stage, and there are many unanswered questions. Although studies have shown consistent links between technology use and sleep, most of these studies are cross-sectional (Bartel & Gradisar, 2017). Experimental studies are more mixed. In one elegant study involving tests of presleep alertness, sleep, and morning functioning in 16 adolescents, 1 hour of screen time before bedtime was not harmful to sleep (Heath et al.,

2014). It certainly remains possible that technology contributes to sleep problems because it increases arousal or because it is so engaging that it can be difficult to turn off by the target bedtime. Another possibility is that technology use is increasing in response to sleeping difficulties (Bartel & Gradisar, 2017). Overall, the link between sleep and technology use will be a rich and important area for future research.

CAFFEINE

People metabolize caffeine at very different rates, owing to substantial individual differences in caffeine metabolizing enzymes. Before making caffeine use a target for intervention, first determine how much of a problem the amount and timing of caffeine use is for the client's sleep.

Abrupt changes in caffeine intake will usually result in unpleasant symptoms, such as headache and fatigue. As such, it is wise to facilitate shifts in the amount and timing of caffeine use *slowly*. Also, warn the client of the possible side effects of reduced intake so they are prepared.

Other clients fall asleep at the beginning of the night soon after a cup of coffee or a glass of cola, possibly because they are very sleep deprived. The homeostatic pressure to sleep is overriding the arousal caused by the caffeine. However, the client may not realize that caffeine has a relatively long half-life. When the homeostatic pressure to sleep has been discharged after a few hours of sleep, the caffeine within the body may contribute to waking in the early hours of the morning and make it very difficult to get back to sleep. Of course, another possibility is that a client is not as sensitive to the arousing effects of caffeine.

NAPPING

In general, napping is discouraged during treatment as it discharges the homeostatic pressure to sleep, making it hard to fall asleep at night and stay asleep during the night. However, if a client is not getting enough total sleep time, we encourage taking a nap before 3:00 P.M. for around 20 minutes. The rationale is that there will be sufficient time between 3:00 P.M. and bedtime to rebuild the homeostatic pressure to sleep. However, keep in mind that there are strong individual differences in the tendency to nap.

Part C. Learning a Wake-Up Routine

Drawing on IPSRT principles, we assist each client in creating a "RISE-UP" routine. The aim is to support regular wake-up times and to help clients who have difficulty waking up because of extended sleep inertia. Sleep inertia is the normal transitional state between sleeping and waking. For most people, this is a period of 5–20 minutes of low arousal, nonoptimal performance on cognitive tasks, grogginess, heavy eyes, sore shoulders, and a feeling of wanting to go back to sleep that resolve relatively quickly. For others, particularly people who meet the diagnostic criteria for depression, bipolar disorder, or schizophrenia, a longer period of sleep inertia up to several hours can be experienced (Kanady & Harvey, 2015).

Following the methods established by Kaplan, Talavera, and Harvey (2016), the first step in this core module is to normalize the unpleasant feelings of sleep inertia on waking. Second, we point out that these unpleasant feelings on waking are typically not a good basis for deciding to stay in bed and snooze. The basic message of this module is that it is usually better to get up and get moving. We recommend selecting from a range of resources in Appendices 1 and 2 that help expand on the rationale for this approach.

Crafting an individualized version of the RISE-UP routine can be very helpful in reaching the goal of getting up at a regular time. The routine employs activity scheduling and goal setting to reinforce getting out of bed. Kaplan and colleagues offer the following initial suggestions:

- Refrain from snoozing.
- Increase activity.
- Shower or wash face and hands.
- Extra sunlight.
- Upbeat music.
- Phone a friend.

The specific components of the RISE-UP should be adapted to the preferences of each client; for example, not all clients like upbeat music on waking. Clients are encouraged to add their own creative ideas for what would help them get out of bed. For example, an older teen rigged a set of pulleys so that all the bedroom lights could go on at once with the pull of a string, which was right beside his bed. This helped motivate him to get up. Another teen created a wake-up playlist on her iPod.

The client should be asked to try the RISE-UP for homework for the coming week. Then session by session we review progress on this module and hone the RISE-UP plan. During these reviews, discussing whether the client has noticed that sleep inertia is worse under any specific circumstances can be informative. For instance, clients might notice sleep inertia worsening under the following circumstances.

1. When they have a difficult day ahead or a day that they are not looking forward to. If so, this is an important insight, as it means that the
sleep obtained is not entirely responsible for the feelings experienced
on waking.
2. When they are sleep deprived or are catching up following a period of
sleep deprivation.
3. When they have irregular sleep–wake schedules.

Note that a primary emphasis for Core Module 1, Parts B and C, is on
establishing wind-down and wake-up routines with an appropriate exposure to
dark and light. The emphasis is on helping the client to establish morning and
evening habits that make use of natural morning light and evening dim light
with client-selected electronic curfews.

Occasionally clients have asked if using an alarm clock to wake up is
unhealthy. We are not aware of any evidence to support this idea. In fact, for
many clients, using an alarm is necessary to avoid sleeping in. Remind the client about the information in the handout (either in Appendix 4 or Appendix
5) associated with Cross-Cutting Module 2 in Chapter 3. In particular, it can
be helpful to remind the client that we typically get lighter stages of sleep in
the morning hours, from which it is relatively easy to wake up. Remind the client that sleep inertia is common on waking, including after the alarm goes off.
Sleep inertia is just the normal transition from sleeping to waking, and very few
people wake up feeling energetic. In other words, experiencing the symptoms
of sleep inertia after waking up is not a signal to turn off the alarm and snooze.
Instead, get up and start the day. The symptoms of sleep inertia will subside.

Core Module 2: Improving Daytime Functioning

The rationale for this module is twofold. First, occasional nights of poor sleep
are inevitable, and therefore we all need skills to cope on the day following a
night of poor sleep. Core Module 2 is designed to help people develop skills to
cope. Second, nighttime and daytime impairment can be at least partly functionally independent (Lichstein et al., 2001; Neitzert Semler & Harvey, 2005).
Thus, TranS-C includes strategies to help clients improve their daytime functioning.

We have observed that clients tend to plan their day around the prior
night's sleep and around their energy levels, which they monitor closely. Many
clients believe that energy progressively dissipates throughout the day and that
the only way to generate more energy is to sleep or rest. Accordingly, many of

our clients work hard to conserve energy after a poor night of sleep. At work, for example, they might prioritize easy (but mundane) activities, such as paperwork and data entry, and avoid meetings and socializing, which might be inherently more energy dependent. The downside of these coping strategies is that the day can be unpleasant, boring, and unproductive. Under such conditions, fatigue and sleepiness are almost inevitable.

Accordingly, this module targets the following unhelpful beliefs: "Energy is increased only by rest or sleep"; "The only way I can feel less tired in the day is to sleep more"; and "I don't have much energy, so I need to take care to conserve it." We typically use a behavioral experiment to demonstrate that *there are many factors, other than sleep, that can influence our energy levels.*

The Energy-Generating Experiment

The core of the module is the energy-generating experiment. Typically this experiment begins by reviewing a diary in which sleep and energy during the day have been tracked daily for 1 week. When we examine the diary together with the client, we point out examples when nighttime sleep was good but energy levels in the day were poor and when nighttime sleep was poor but energy levels during the day were good. This review provides an opportunity to introduce the following idea: "Well, that's really interesting. So if sleep doesn't fully account for how you feel during the day, then there must be other things that can account for it." Together, we brainstorm possibilities and write them down (e.g., "the job I had to do that day was boring or stressful," "I had a fight with my girlfriend"). We then use these possibilities as the basis of the energy-generating experiment. We recommend saying, "I wonder if you would be willing to try an experiment with me in which we do the opposite of these things and see what happens to your energy level?"

As we set up the experiment, we explicitly say that that we are testing the following beliefs: "Energy is increased only by rest or sleep" and "I don't have much energy, so I need to take care to conserve it." The specific way that the belief is stated ideally incorporates the client's own words. The experiment itself can take various forms.

Option 1

Compare 2 days of doing "what you usually do" when you get tired (e.g., taking a nap) to 2 days of doing something different. The alternative might be very new to the client, and so brainstorm with the client exactly what the alternative would be. The list will typically include activities like getting exercise, going out into the sunlight, and visiting with a friend. We also devise a way to collect data on the client's observations as soon as possible after the two conditions. For example, we might ask the client to text the therapist a rating from 1 ("very low energy") to 10 ("very high energy") of how he or she felt after each activity. Or we might ask the client to write his or her rating down on a form specifically devised for this experiment.

Option 2

A version of this experiment can be done in the session by asking the client to rate his or her energy level on a scale of 1 to 10. You, the therapist, should rate your energy too. Then together with the client, do an activity, such as go for a walk outside or walk or run up and down stairs. If the client has restricted mobility, do chair exercises together. Chair exercises are body workouts that are done from the support of a chair, such as seated jumping jacks or abs twisters. After, both should rerate their energy levels and discuss their experience and draw conclusions.

Option 3

Design an experiment that unfolds over 2 days. On the first day spend one 3-hour block *conserving* energy, and then one 3-hour block *using* energy. The following day do the experiment again, but in the reverse order. After each 3-hour block, the client rates his or her fatigue, mood, and coping on a 1–10 scale. Prior to the experiment, through careful questioning, endeavor to understand what conserving energy means for the client. Examples include avoiding socializing with colleagues, setting work tasks at a slow pace, attempting only mundane tasks, not going out for lunch with work friends, and not returning phone calls. Also, spend time in the session brainstorming strategies for using energy. These might include going for a 10-minute walk, returning all phone calls, arranging to have a coffee with a colleague, getting on top of paperwork, going to the water cooler to get a drink, or walking to a local shop to buy a magazine or snack.

These experiments typically vividly illustrate our belief that there are factors other than sleep that influence energy levels. More specifically, clients can learn through completing these experiments that there are many factors that influence energy levels during the day. They usually conclude that daytime energy levels are elastic and can be expanded quite easily. This view contrasts with their original, unhelpful view that energy levels progressively diminish throughout the day. Clients are then well positioned to start developing a list of

---

BOX 4.1. Managing Daytime Tiredness

Actions that can be taken during the day to *increase* the adverse effects of poor sleep	Actions that can be taken during the day to *decrease* the adverse effects of poor sleep
• Think or dwell on feeling worthless • Cancel social outings • Think about how bad I feel • Take the afternoon off work and take a long nap • Think about and plan for getting a good night's sleep tonight	• Run the dogs • Take a walk not drive • Catch negative thoughts and challenge them • Engage in more challenging and attention consuming activities, such as going to the gym or arranging an outing with a friend

---

"energy-generating" and "energy-sapping" activities to better manage daytime tiredness (see Box 4.1 for an example). Week by week continue to work on ways to improve functioning in the daytime and to develop the menu of options for coping after a poor night of sleep.

Tip

The evidence that accrues during this experiment should be revisited in future sessions to reinforce the experience. Furthermore, we ensure that the client overtly adopts the energy-generating activities when feeling tired in day-to-day life. If so, they will need to be supported with practice between sessions and discussion during the session (e.g., "In what ways did you manage to generate energy?"; "What do you think went wrong?"). Retrospective experiments can also be useful—for example: "Can you think of a day after a poor night's sleep when you became energized sometime during the day, say, if you had to attend an exciting event?"

Countering a Belief That Tiredness Is Completely Due to Medication

Some clients who are taking sedating medications believe that these medications are entirely responsible for their daytime tiredness and that they have no control over how they feel. We suggest trying the following exercise, and start by saying, "Let's think about all the things that might contribute to your feeling tired in the day." Medications will be on this list. Other items that might be listed include not getting enough exercise, feeling bored with work, eating too much sugar and junk food, and not having enough social time. Then draw a circle on a white board or on a blank sheet of paper and say, "OK, let's think about this together. Among these many contributors to feeling tired in the day, what proportion of your daytime tiredness might be due to not getting enough exercise?" The client might allocate 20%. Then start dividing the circle into "pie pieces," carving out a slice that accounts for approximately 20%. Label it "not enough exercise." Then do the same for all the other contributing factors, adding in the proportion of the pie due to the sedating medicines toward the end. Finally, initiate a discussion along the lines of "So isn't this interesting? It appears that there are some modifiable contributors to feeling tired in the day, such as not getting enough exercise, staying indoors all day, and feeling isolated from friends and family. Given this, would you be interested in trying an experiment where perhaps we can increase social contact, get a bit more exercise, and spend some time outdoors and see whether this helps?" This short exercise tends to shift the client's perspective and be hopeful about their ability to improve their daytime functioning, while continuing to adhere to the medications.

Experimenting with Attention

Attentional processes can subtly interfere with daytime energy. We introduce this idea to clients by explaining:

> "If you are very concerned about something, it makes sense that you would be on the lookout for it and be particularly alert to anything that is relevant to your concern. In a similar way, people with sleep problems are on the lookout for signs of their sleep problem, particularly throughout the day. However, being on the lookout or in 'alert mode' can end up fueling problems. Let me give an example of a typical situation to see whether it resonates with you. Immediately on waking Sally would monitor her body to see whether it felt sufficiently rested. She nearly always noticed that her muscles felt sore and tired and that her eyes felt heavy. She'd then think 'Oh no! I didn't get enough sleep last night.' This would make her feel sad and also anxious as she wondered how she would cope with the day ahead. During the day, Sally would monitor for feelings of tiredness, checking how clear her head felt and how heavy her legs felt when she walked up the stairs to her office. She would also be on the lookout for lapses in performance during the work day."

Ask clients whether they engage in monitoring during the day and whether they have predictions about the impact of this on their daytime energy. Then consider whether to do one of the following experiments:

1. During session time, go for a walk together. First, rate how you each feel on a 0–10 tiredness and fatigue scale. Then spend 5 minutes walking, while internally monitoring how the body feels, paying particular attention to signs of tiredness and fatigue. After 5 minutes, rate how you both feel afterward. Then spend the next 5 minutes focusing externally on the trees, flowers, and sky, and rerate how you each feel on a 0–10 tiredness and fatigue scale. Go back to the office to debrief.

2. Between sessions, suggest that the client experiment with a weekend hike. He or she would start by spending 30 minutes asking and answering questions like "How do my legs feel right now?"; "How does my torso feel right now?"; "What about my shoulders and head—how do they feel?" The client then rates (on a 0–10 scale in a small notebook) his or her level of tiredness, energy, and enjoyment of the walk. He or she then spends 30 minutes asking and answering questions like "What can I see?"; "Is the scenery pleasant?"; "Are the wildflowers out?" The client then rerates the previous levels.

The essential feature of these experiments is having clients experience turning their attention outward toward "smelling the flowers," "getting out of their heads and getting lost in the world around them," and in "turning the radar off." A saying that we often mention is "If you look for trouble, you find trouble." Instead, clients get to experience the relief and energy that comes from redirecting their attention.

What to Do If the Client Is Sleepy in the Session

We have found several helpful strategies for working with clients who are sleepy during the session.

• Consider conducting part of the session standing up. We tried this recently with a teen who was sleepy, depressed, and unengaged. When the therapist observed that the teen was struggling with sleepiness, she suggested that they both stand up for part of the session. The therapist then stood up, and the teen followed. After 3 minutes the teen sat down, and the therapist followed. This small shift was surprisingly effective for engaging the teen and reducing sleepiness.

• Cover some of the session content with videos. Video presentations can be more engaging and help clients remain more alert. A list of helpful videos is included in Appendix 2.

• Suggest to clients that you both do an energy-generating activity of their choice. Some adolescent clients have selected push-ups or jumping jacks. Others have selected a yoga sequence. We have also used chair exercises for clients with restricted mobility. This in-session behavioral experiment is best set up as part of the energy- generating experiment by asking the client to rate his or her current energy levels on a 1 ("no energy") to 10 ("maximum energy") scale before and after the experiment. Volunteer your own ratings.

• Increase the amount of guided discovery to help to keep the client engaged and promote processing and understanding of the material.

• Use thought experiments by asking "What do you think would happen if . . . ?"

• Elicit the client's own experiences to illustrate key points.

• Create regular written summaries of the main points covered in every session. This is a core CBT skill. Asking the client to write the summaries themselves is ideal and will help keep the client alert. But don't hesitate to write the summary yourself if a client is reluctant.

• Set up a "behavioral prescription" (similar to a physician's prescription) in the form of preprinted sheets that are personalized with bedtimes, wake times, and any nap times.

Core Module 3: Correcting Unhelpful Sleep-Related Beliefs

Holding unhelpful beliefs about sleep is common and includes beliefs such as "Sleep is a waste of time"; "Everyone except me sleep. 8 hours a night and wakes up feeling bright and alert"; "It's not normal to feel tired and experience lapses in memory and concentration at times during the day"; "I can train myself to get less sleep." In Chapter 2 we described the DBAS, an assessment of unhelpful beliefs about sleep relevant to insomnia. In addition, you will likely spot additional unhelpful beliefs about sleep held by your clients as you get to know them.

There is a compelling rationale for including a focus on unhelpful beliefs about sleep as a core module. Several studies show that a reduction in unhelpful beliefs about sleep both before and after treatment for insomnia is associated with persistent, enduring improvements in sleep once the treatment has ended (Edinger et al., 2001; Morin et al., 2002).

Keep in mind that this module needs to be adapted to the clinical realities of certain disorders. For instance, one DBAS item is "I am worried that if I go for 1 or 2 nights without sleep I may have a "nervous breakdown." While this *is* an unhelpful belief for most clients with insomnia, sleep deprivation in bipolar disorder *can* be dangerous because it can trigger a manic episode. As such, clients with bipolar disorder are often anxious about their sleep, in part because they are aware that sleep loss can herald relapse (Harvey, Schmidt, Scarna, Semler, & Goodwin, 2005). Since anxiety is antithetical to sleep (Espie, 2002), in these cases we change the focus to working with bedtime worry, rumination, and anxiety (discussed in Chapter 5, Optional Module 4), rather than altering the belief.

We use education, guided discovery, and individualized experiments to address unhelpful beliefs about sleep (Ree & Harvey, 2004). The experiments should be tailored to each client, and new experiments can be devised to address other beliefs held by the client. Several examples are offered below and are also described elsewhere (Harvey & Eidelman, 2011; Harvey & Talbot, 2011). The energy-generating experiments that target unhelpful beliefs about daytime tiredness can also be beneficial and have already been described in Core Module 2.

An Experiment to Counter a Belief in Control over Sleep

Another commonly held belief is "I will lose control over my ability to sleep. I have to try really hard to sleep and get control back." A useful experiment to counter this belief involves having the client do everything possible to control his or her sleep on the first night; on the second night, the client drops all attempts to sleep. Before embarking on this experiment, it is very important to specifically define how your client controls his or her sleep and explain how to drop these attempts at control. Efforts to control sleep will likely vary from person to person, and it is important to outline them in some detail before the experiment is attempted. Ask clients to predict the outcome of the experiment. A typical prediction made by a client is that "unless I try very hard to get to sleep, I will have a terrible night of sleep." The daily sleep diary can be used to measure the outcome, paying particular attention to the amount of time it took the client to get to sleep and how long he or she was awake over the course of the night.

After the experiment, clients typically conclude that the more they try to control their sleep, the more out of control they are. In other words, actively trying to control sleep makes the situation worse. This experiment is also a good basis for having a discussion about sleep being an automatic biological process that does not need to be controlled. We also discuss the research conducted by Niall Broomfield and Colin Espie showing that attempts to control sleep actually exacerbate and perpetuate insomnia (Broomfield & Espie, 2005). Finally, we share the interesting observation by Espie (2002) that good sleepers, if asked what they do to fall asleep, are confused by the question and can't report on any specific behavior. In other words, sleep is a passive and effortless state (Espie, 2002). We also explain that good sleepers struggle to stay awake, whereas individuals with insomnia struggle to go to sleep. In other words, good sleepers fall asleep because they can no longer stay awake—not because they are trying to sleep. In short, sleep is an involuntary process. You can, within limits, force yourself to stay awake, but you can never force yourself to fall asleep.

A Survey Experiment on How Others Sleep

This next experiment is adapted from David M. Clark's research on the anxiety disorders (Clark et al., 2006). The goal of the *survey experiment* is to broaden the client's perspective on what constitutes normal sleep. By collaboratively devising and administering a survey to a set of individuals who are close to the client's age, the client gathers data about the variety of sleep experiences obtained by others. Additionally, he or she might include questions that elicit ideas for coping strategies. Prior to conducting this experiment, we suggest revisiting the client's responses to the DBAS (Morin, 1993). For each item rated higher than halfway on the rating scale, prepare a survey question designed to help the client obtain corrective information. Also, go through your notes for all past sessions to identify other unhelpful beliefs the client has. Before the session prepare drafts of survey questions designed to obtain data on these issues.

We introduce this experiment by asking the client how he or she developed ideas about sleep. Does he or she have some ideas about how good sleepers sleep? Does he or she have some curiosity about these ideas? Many clients are eager to learn more about the way other people sleep and to approach the issue in a scientific manner.

Then introduce the survey.

"One of the components of this treatment that we have found to be very effective is for us to collaborate on creating and administering a survey. There are many things we can learn from it.

- "Conducting a survey can be a way to get advice from good sleepers about why they sleep so well.
- "It can also remind us how well good sleepers really sleep. Often the people who come for treatment have forgotten what being a good sleeper is.
- "The survey also helps ensure our beliefs about sleep are data based. Most people develop their ideas about sleep from magazine articles or a parent or on the basis of their own experience.

"Would you be interested in devising a survey together and administering it to people in your age group? We focus on people around your age because sleep changes so much depending on age, and we want these data to be relevant and applicable to you. Here are some questions we have found to be helpful in the past. [Show the questions you have designed prior to the session.] So what you and I need to do together now is to decide which of these questions to include, whether we want to reword any of them, and whether there are additional questions you want to use."

We design the survey collaboratively with the client in the treatment session within an online survey delivery system (e.g., *www.surveymonkey.com*). See Box 4.2 for a completed sample survey with questions that might be included. Typically the client will try to collect 10 or more responses, and the therapist will try to collect some responses as well. We always try to include people within 5 years on either side of the client's age. This respects sleep-related changes with age. For example, it wouldn't make sense for a 70-year-old client to include responses from a 20-year-old given the differences between the sleep experience of those in their 70s and those in their 20s. This is also an opportunity to discuss survey design more generally and the sources of potential bias, noting that the results will be more valid and less likely to be skewed by unusual responders if the sample size is large. These are helpful seeds to plant in case the survey ends up consisting of a small skewed sample.

In the session that follows, examine the results of the survey together and discuss the conclusions the client draws. See Box 4.2 for an example of a collated survey and the conclusions that were drawn. The survey reveals that the majority of people have some trouble with sleep when feeling stressed and feel tired when they wake up and again after lunch, that most people have trouble sleeping at least some of the time, and that it is unrealistic to expect 8 hours sleep every night. As a consequence of these discoveries, the client's expectations of sleep and daytime tiredness may shift, and anxiety about attaining "perfect" sleep is reduced. Strategies for coping with poor sleep are also generated.

BOX 4.2. Example of a Survey Experiment
(Age Range: 50–60 Years)

1. On average, how long does it take you to fall asleep?

   0–10 minutes = 2 responses
   11–20 minutes = 5 responses
   21–30 minutes = 12 responses
   31–40 minutes = 5 responses
   41–50 minutes = 1 response
   51–60 minutes = 1 response
   61+ minutes = no responses

   Conclusion: **Many respondents take a long time to fall asleep (i.e., 20–30 minutes). Very few people fall asleep as soon as their head hits the pillow. This is good to know. My husband falls asleep as soon as his head hits the pillow, so I thought I was abnormal for taking 20–30 minutes to fall to sleep.**

2. How many hours of sleep do you typically get?

   4 hours = no responses
   5 hours = 1 response
   6 hours = 2 responses
   7 hours = 9 responses
   8 hours = 10 responses
   9 hours = 4 responses
   10 hours = no responses

   Conclusion: **Most of the respondents sleep between 7 and 8 hours per night. It's interesting to see how many adults are getting less than 8 hours on a typical night. Perhaps I don't need to be quite so focused on getting 8 hours every night.**

3. If you got less than your ideal amount of sleep, how many hours could you get by with (per night) for 2 nights in a row?

   3 hours = 1 response
   4 hours = 4 responses
   5 hours = 9 responses
   6 hours = 12 responses
   7 hours = No responses
   8 hours = No responses

   Conclusion: **5 hours of sleep seems to be the average amount of sleep people can get by with. I thought I needed 8 hours every night to get by.**

4. Most people wake up in the night. How many times do you wake up, even if just for a few seconds?

   0 times = 3 responses

   1–2 times = 16 responses

   3–4 times = 7 responses

   Conclusion: **I thought there was something wrong with me because I wake up 1–2 times per night. It's interesting to see that most people wake up during the night between 1 and 3 times. I guess that waking in the night is normal for adults.**

5. Do you ever have times you feel tired and lethargic in the day?

   Yes = 23 responses

   No = 3 responses

   Conclusion: **Most people feel tired during the day. Again, I thought there was something wrong with me because I often feel tired.**

Experiments on the Perception of Sleep

It is not uncommon for people with sleep and circadian rhythm problems to believe they get less sleep than they actually do as measured by objective assessments (Harvey & Tang, 2012). This is another important perception to address because it can contribute to anxiety about sleep, which in turn, contributes to poor sleep.

In all sessions we suggest being alert to natural opportunities to explore this topic. For example, the client might say:

> "Something weird happened last night. I honestly thought I hardly slept at all but when I told my wife over breakfast this morning she laughed and said that I was fast asleep, and breathing heavily, all night. She knew this because she wasn't feeling well and was awake a lot. You know, I believe her because she's very supportive of me and wouldn't say I was asleep if I wasn't."

If this happens, seize the opportunity to explore this experience by asking, "What sense do you make of this?" If the client doesn't mention the possibility that he or she misperceived sleep, offer the information that sleep is incredibly difficult to reliably perceive because sleep onset is defined by the absence of memories. Also, give examples of your own difficulties in perceiving sleep.

- *Example A*: "I have sometimes had the experience of meaning to nap on a Sunday afternoon for just 10 to 20 minutes but then wake up 2 hours later unable to believe how much time has passed."
- *Example B*: "Particularly vivid to me is that when flying from London to Sydney I thought I was asleep for 2–3 hours. But when I woke up I was disappointed to learn that I had only been asleep for 20 minutes."

Ask clients if they have their own examples.

There are three behavioral experiments that can be used to correct the perception of sleep. First, add a question to the sleep diary to assess daytime energy (e.g., on a scale from 1 ("no energy") to 10 ("lots of energy"). When the client returns to review the sleep diary, draw attention to those nights when the client records very poor sleep in the diary but reasonable daytime functioning. Ask "What sense do you make of this?" This typically begins as discussion wherein education about perceptions of sleep can be offered. Introduce the points previously covered.

Second, for clients with many episodes of waking after sleep onset each night, we ask the client to keep a golf counter under his or her pillow and to press the counter each time he or she wakes up. In the morning on waking ask the client to record the number on the golf counter. Typically this will yield a vast reduction in the estimates of episodes of waking throughout the night. Third, if actigraphy is available, we teach clients to download and read their actigraphy data and compare it to their sleep diary data. They can then discover for themselves the tendency to overestimate the time they take to get to sleep at the beginning of the night and to underestimate their total sleep time. Compared to simply providing education about the perception of sleep, this procedure improved the accuracy of clients' subjective perceptions and reduced sleep-related anxiety and preoccupation (Tang & Harvey, 2006). The Appendix 10 handout summarizes the information on our perception of sleep.

Core Module 4: Maintenance of Behavior Change

The goal of this module is to consolidate gains and prepare for setbacks, using an individualized summary of what the client has learned and his or her achievements. In every session throughout the entire treatment we keep an eye out for opportunities to promote the maintenance of behavior change (as described in Core Module 3). Then in the second to last session we start to prepare in earnest by reviewing and charting the client's progress using the weekly data from the sleep diary, checking on goal attainment, identifying specific problem areas that need more attention, and summarizing the learning that has taken place over the course of treatment. The questions we use to help guide this process are in Box 4.3. We ask the client to complete these questions for homework before the final session. The therapist also completes the same questions for the final session. It is always interesting to compare the client and therapist versions.

For youth (and other clients who might be interested), we co-create a summary video of the top five tips on how to improve sleep. An example of a 13-year-old's list of top tips is presented in Box 4.4. Note that this teen actually generated eight tips because she was so excited about her newly acquired sleep knowledge! The video might take the form of a commercial for other people or an interview with a journalist (the therapist plays the role of journalist). We record the video in the last session as a way to consolidate learning and treatment gains. The video is just for the client's benefit; no one else will see it unless he or she decides to share it. If your client doesn't want to make a video, he or she might consider drawing a comic strip or writing a song—any activity that will help consolidate learning. Feel free to be creative. We believe that linking a summary of everything that the client has absorbed in the course of TranS-C to a novel task will create a stronger learning experience and promote better recall of the main treatment points.

BOX 4.3. Questions Used to Summarize Progress and Prevent Relapse

1. "How did the problem develop?"
2. "What kept it going?"
3. "What did you learn during therapy about how to overcome the problem?"
4. "What were your most unhelpful thoughts and beliefs? What are the alternatives to these?"
5. "What were your most unhelpful behaviors? What are alternatives to these?"
6. "How will you build on what you have learned? What do you think are the most important things to remember in order to keep your progress going?"
7. "Setbacks are inevitable. What steps will you take if you have a setback?"

**BOX 4.4. A 13-Year-Old Female's Top Tips
for Improving Sleep**

---

1. Melatonin makes you sleepy, and light stops melatonin from being released.
2. Circadian rhythm is important because it is the body's natural rhythm for sleep.
3. Wake up at the same time every day.
4. Naps make sleep pressure go down, because your sleep pressure has to start all over again after a nap.
5. Conditioning: don't do anything in bed, but sleep. Don't worry in bed.
6. Worry and excitement keep you awake.
7. If you can't get to sleep, get out of bed and read with a flashlight.
8. Staying up later and waking up later on weekends gives you jet lag every single week.

There are several other points to make in this final phase.

• It is unrealistic to expect to sleep well every single night. It is much more realistic to expect that there will be some periods when progress feels very strong, and other periods when sleep is more variable. We suggest that when the clients go through a period of more variable sleep they try not to become overly discouraged or concerned, but rather return to the material we have covered in the therapy sessions. They should think through what they need to do to get steady progress back on track.

• With the client, we identify high-risk triggers to sleep problems, such as negative emotional states (e.g., stress, daily hassles) and positive emotional states (e.g., anticipation of a trip, a change of schedules) and make a plan for how the client can manage these triggers.

• Remind clients of strategies for coping with inevitable problems, such as stay calm; there is no need to panic, it just makes things worse; analyze the antecedents or precipitating circumstances; review the materials collected from treatment and make a plan that applies to the current circumstances; ask for further help.

• Emphasize the "long view" with clients—in other words, the important focus is not how well you slept last night, but rather, how well you slept the last week or month.

CHAPTER 5

TranS-C Optional Modules

The seven optional modules of TranS-C that are covered in this chapter are used less commonly than the core modules and depend on the needs of each client. For each optional module we briefly describe when to administer the module, the background and rationale for the module, and the steps involved in delivering the module.

Optional Module 1: Improving Sleep Efficiency

When to Use Optional Module 1

Optional Module 1 is usually delivered starting around Session 4 if a client's sleep efficiency (SE) as recorded in the sleep diary is less than 85% on average across 1 week (adjust this value to 80% for older adults). SE is calculated for each day of the daily sleep diary by dividing TST by TIB and multiplying this value by 100. Then the average of the SE values for each day becomes the SE value for the week.

Background

Sleeping efficiently is a dimension of the sleep health framework. It refers to the ability to sleep for a large percentage of the time spent in bed. It is indicated by the ease of falling asleep at the beginning of the night and the ease of return-ing to sleep after awakenings during the night. This dimension is one of the six core dimensions of sleep health because of the evidence that sleep inefficiency is associated with increased mortality, coronary heart disease, metabolic syn-drome, hypertension, and depression (Buysse, 2014).

The content of this module is based on the extensive insomnia literature showing the effectiveness of two components of CBT-I for improving SE—stimulus control and sleep restriction (Morin et al., 2006). The theoretical basis for these interventions is that maladaptive conditioning has taken place, whereby the bed or bedroom has become paired with being awake and anxious about not sleeping. Stimulus control and sleep restriction are designed to break the nonsleep associations and rebuild the association between the bed and consolidated sleep.

Interventions

Stimulus Control

Developed by Richard Bootzin and colleagues (Bootzin, Epstein, & Wood, 1991), stimulus control involves a series of four specific behavioral recommen-dations. The recommendations, along with suggestions for introducing them, are outlined below.

GO TO BED ONLY WHEN SLEEPY

The goal of this recommendation is to reestablish the association between the bed and sleep. Clients are asked to only go to bed and stay in bed when they feel sleepy and when they are close to falling to sleep. It is important to teach the distinction between "sleepiness" and "tiredness" and to encourage people to wait until they feel sleepy before getting into bed. By this point in the treat-ment you will have assisted the client in creating an individualized wind-down (Core Module 1, Part B) to promote sleepiness at the appropriate time of the day. We also like to point out that sleep is not a voluntary process. If it were, we could just decide to go to sleep whenever we wanted. That's obviously not the case. We can only sleep when our brain is *ready* for sleep—when it has built up enough "sleep drive" from a long period of prior wakefulness. Sleepiness is the indicator that we have built up enough sleep drive. Sleeping becomes more dif-ficult and less achievable the harder we try. So if the client is not sleepy, there's no point in trying to force sleep. He or she should just stay up a bit longer until the sleep drive is stronger.

For some clients, this recommendation is modified to reduce the risk of engagement in goal-seeking and rewarding behaviors (Johnson, 2005) that could further reduce sleep opportunity. Some clients need to be away from technology and in darkness or dim light before they start to feel sleepy. Also, there is evidence that people diagnosed with bipolar disorder are particularly sensitive to light (Barbini et al., 2005; Benedetti, Colombo, Barbini, Campori, & Smeraldi, 2001; Sit, Wisner, Hanusa, Stull, & Terman, 2007). In these cases, going to bed and turning off the lights may be needed in order to feel sleepy. Another approach would be to work on reducing evening light, or even wearing sunglasses or welding glasses. This modification of traditional stimulus control should be given a trial, closely monitoring the sleep diary to determine if it was helpful.

GET OUT OF BED IF UNABLE TO FALL ASLEEP

Because time spent awake in bed can often be associated with worry, rumination, and escalating arousal, clients are asked to leave their beds if they are not falling asleep within 15–20 minutes. We often use a blank sheet of paper to draw a vicious cycle: wakefulness → frustration → worry → arousal → wakefulness. We point out that getting out of bed interrupts that cycle.

Clock watching is discouraged given the evidence that it increases anxiety about sleep and the difficulty of accurately perceiving the amount of sleep (Tang et al., 2007). Instead, clients are encouraged to use their "felt-sense" to estimate the time. Reassure the client that their best guess is good enough. They are asked to remain up and return to bed only when they feel sleepy.

Collaboratively work out a plan for what the client will do when he or she is out of bed. Ideally he or she should go into another room and engage in a quiet activity that is relaxing and calming, such as journaling, meditating, reading a magazine or book, listening to music, doing a crossword puzzle, or something else that is nonarousing. We encourage clients to place warm clothing by their bed to increase their comfort. Keeping the lights as dim as possible is a high priority, as our circadian clocks are especially sensitive to light in the middle of the night.

Potentially stimulating activities such as web browsing, watching certain TV programs, catching up on email, and cleaning the house are discouraged. The client is asked to return to bed only when he or she feels sleepy and to repeat these steps as often as necessary throughout the night. Any time the client wakes up and is awake for more than 20 minutes, he or she should get out of bed and engage in a quiet activity. When the client does start to feel sleepy, he or she should head back to bed. It's important to make the association that bed equals sleep!

Many of our clients live in studio apartments or single rooms, or they share a room. In these situations we suggest that clients find an alternate place when getting out of bed, such as a chair or a pillow on the floor. For clients who are bedbound, try differentiating sleep–wake periods with lying down versus sitting up in bed.

KEEP THE BEDROOM FOR SLEEP AND SEX

We want to train the brain to think that bed equals sleep and being awake equals being somewhere else. Many people with sleep problems have unintentionally taught their brain that the bed equals the place to do a lot of frustrated tossing and turning. This recommendation involves removing all sleep-incompatible activities (watching TV, eating, completing homework, holding conflictual discussions with a family member) from the bed and bedroom. Remind clients that time in bed spent awake watching TV weakens the association between the bed and sleep. Of course, the increased availability of portable technology has increased the challenge associated with this recommendation. As addressed in Core Module 1, Part B, we work with the client to create an electronic curfew or, if that is not possible, take harm-reduction measures.

DISCOURAGE NAPPING

Napping discharges homeostatic pressure to sleep (see Chapter 1 for a review of the two-process model of sleep), making it more difficult to fall asleep or stay asleep at night. This is especially true for naps that occur in the late afternoon or evening. Although these naps feel helpful in the short term, they can make it more difficult to fall asleep later that night, disrupt the circadian rhythm, and perpetuate long-term insomnia. If clients really need to nap, we recommend scheduling the nap for before 3:00 P.M. and for only 20 minutes to ensure that the homeostatic pressure to sleep can rebuild in time for bedtime. The energy-generating experiment described in Core Module 2 can be adapted to help people gain firsthand experience with the problems associated with naps.

Sleep Restriction

As developed by Arthur Spielman and colleagues (Spielman et al., 1987), the basic idea of sleep restriction is that TIB should be limited to maximize the sleep drive and strengthen the association between the bed and sleeping. This approach begins with a reduction in the amount of time spent in bed so that TIB becomes equivalent to the time the client estimates he or she spends sleeping. However, note that Spielman, Yang, and Glovinsky (2011) have recommended a lower limit of 5 hours per night, a recommendation that we suggest revising for certain client groups, as discussed later in the section on "Cautions."

Here are the steps for administering sleep restriction: Calculate TST, TIB, and SE based on the prior week's sleep diary. Recall that SE is defined as TST divided by TIB, then multiplied by 100 to equal a percentage. For example, on reviewing the pretreatment sleep diary for a client who meets diagnostic criteria for depression, it became apparent that this client slept an average of 6 hours per night over the week and spent an average of 9½ hours in bed. SE for the week will be $6 \div 9.5 \times 100$, or 63%. The goal over the course of TranS-C is to increase SE to more than 85%. In this case we would set a "sleep window" equal to the prior week's TST (6 hours), choosing a preferred bedtime and rise time with the client. We assess whether the client has a preference for waking up earlier or going to bed later and co-create a plan to facilitate the client's preference. Session-by-session progress is evaluated. As soon as SE reaches 85%, the client and therapist gradually expand the window (e.g., by 30 minutes per week) toward the optimal sleep time.

One strategy that is particularly helpful is asking questions to help the client derive the "TIB prescription." For example:

> "OK, let's start with a time that makes sense for you to wake up every day. [Assess the client's preference.] All right, now your diary indicates that you're getting about 5 hours of sleep on average, right? OK, so let's figure out your bedtime by working backward. What time is 5 hours before X? [Help the client do the calculation.] So, your bedtime should really be Y. How does that sound? [Listen to the client's response.] If you really want to get a solid block of sleep, you should go to bed at Y. Remember, we don't want you to get less sleep—we just want to get a solid block of sleep, and push the wakefulness to the beginning and end of the night. But, just to show you I'm not being cruel or unreasonable, let's give you another 30 minutes—after all, nobody can sleep 100% of the time in bed. So that would make your bedtime Y–30 minutes."

The following analogy is very useful for explaining sleep restriction.

> "Imagine we have a tall glass of water. It's a deep, tight column of water. Now imagine if we took that glass of water and poured it into a bathtub. What would happen? The water would spread out to cover as much space as possible, and it would get very shallow. Your sleep now is kind of like the water in the bathtub—shallow and broken up. Limiting your time in bed is like putting the water back in the glass—a deep, solid column. The amount of water is the same in either case—it's just a question of being spread out versus being consolidated. Do you think your sleep would be more satisfactory if it were spread across a longer time in bed,

or experienced as a more solid block? I'm not saying you should get less sleep—I'm just saying that by spending less time in bed your sleep may be more continuous and less broken up. And most people find that to be more restful and satisfying."

CAUTIONS

All of these recommended strategies can cause some short-term sleep deprivation and should be delivered with great care. There are several types of clients, among others you may encounter, for whom adaptation is indicated. The first are those who drive or operate tools for work. This module may be contraindicated for these clients given the known effect of sleep deprivation in driving ability. The second group is made up of clients with a severe mental illness like bipolar disorder. There is evidence that sleep deprivation can trigger a relapse (e.g., Colombo, Benedetti, Barbini, Campori, & Smeraldi, 1999). Hence, to minimize the risk of relapse from sleep deprivation, we recommend that TIB be restricted to no less than 6½ hours per night.

Optional Module 2: Reducing TIB

When to Use Optional Module 2

If TIB (including daytime naps) is greater than 9–10 hours for adults or 10½–11½ hours for youth, on average, across 1 week of the daily sleep diary, we typically deliver Optional Module 2 starting around Session 4. TIB is determined by averaging the data in the daily sleep diary.

Background

Therapists who are new to sleep medicine are often surprised to learn that getting *too much sleep* and spending *too much time in bed* can be problems. As discussed in Chapter 1, sleep duration and SE are two of the dimensions of the sleep health framework (Buysse, 2014). Together, these dimensions emphasize seeking the middle road for sleep duration and TIB; both too little and too much are problematic. This TranS-C module is focused on clients, often with a comorbid mental illness, who often spend too much time in bed. It is important, though, to distinguish spending too much time in bed and feeling sleepy during the day from narcolepsy and hypersomnolence disorder. The latter two disorders require a referral to a medically trained sleep specialist, who will conduct a thorough assessment and treatment. Unfortunately, distinguishing hypersomnolence disorder from the behavioral condition of spending too much time in bed can be very challenging. As presented in Table 2.2, hypersomnolence disorder is characterized by good SE at night, by actual sleepiness and napping during the day, by the desire to engage in more activities, and by less-severe psychiatric symptoms. On the other hand, the behavioral condition of spending too much time in bed is characterized by poor SE at night, low motivation, anergia, and fatigue rather than by actual sleepiness; by a lack of motivation to engage in activities; and by more severe psychiatric symptoms. This latter condition is the focus of the current discussion.

Spending an excessive amount of time in bed is an important treatment target for several reasons (Kaplan & Harvey, 2009). First, it impairs the client's ability to live life fully and makes it difficult to for him or her to fully engage with work, family, and friends. Second, it is associated with more emotional disturbance, unhappiness and interpersonal problems, more substance abuse, excessive daytime sleepiness, and impairment in daily activities and in the level of productivity (Kaplan et al., 2011). Third, it is possible that it will have an adverse impact on health, because the human body has evolved to spend two-thirds of each day in the light and being active. Finally, as described in Optional Module 1, too much time in bed is typically associated with fragmented sleep, poor sleep efficiency, and reports of not feeling rested on waking.

Interventions

The overall goal of this TranS-C module is to reduce TIB to a reasonable amount and improve SE. Two factors determine the amount of time that is reasonable. The first is the age of the client. Keep in mind that youth and young adults require 8½–9½ hours of sleep per night, adults in the middle years require 7–8 hours of sleep per night, and older adults require around 7 hours of sleep per night. Second, consider that some medications have sedating side effects. If a medication your client is taking is sedating, we suggest adjusting the goals, for example, by allowing for an extra hour in bed.

Education about Sleep Inertia

Remind the client about the education they received on sleep inertia (covered in Core Module 1, Part C). The experience of sleep inertia can be very unpleasant, and avoiding it can be a key reason why people stay in bed well into the daytime hours. A common belief is that *getting more sleep will reduce sleep inertia*. However, there's evidence for the opposite belief—when we spend too much time in bed, we often feel worse.

*Revisiting the Wind-Down and RISE-UP
(Core Module 1, Parts B and C)*

Continue to emphasize regularity and minimizing the fluctuation in the sleep–wake schedule across the nights of the week and to encourage strategies to help with getting up each morning. These modules support reducing TIB.

Assessing Why the Client Spends a Lot of TIB

Common reasons include beliefs about sleep being curative, avoidance, and having nothing to get up for. See Box 5.1 for a sample list of pros and cons for oversleeping generated by one client with bipolar disorder.

Reducing TIB by 30–60 Minutes per Week

The treatment principle guiding this next step is the same as the one that has already been described for sleep restriction in Optional Module 1. If the client is willing to take the sleep-restriction approach, that is terrific! In our experience, we have usually needed to take a slower approach, which is akin to Ken Lichstein's description of sleep compression (Lichstein, 1988). We set a long-range goal for the amount of nighttime sleep the client would like to get, and we aim to achieve this goal by the end of treatment. The short-term, or week-by-week goals for the night, are to slowly reduce TIB at each session, usually in

---

BOX 5.1. The Pros and Cons of Oversleeping from a Patient with Bipolar Disorder

Pros	Cons
• Sleep is healing, renewing. • If I sleep 14 hours a day, my body must need it. • Sleep will help to heal my mind and reduce manic, racing thoughts. • It kills time.	• Fewer hours in a day to do things. • I want to go back to work and feel productive. • Relationships: when I sleep so much I can't keep a girlfriend or friends. • Makes me sluggish and depressed.

30–60 minute increments per week. Many clients return to the session, after a first try, and have achieved the goal on only 1 or a few nights that week. It is important to recognize that achievement and work through the obstacles the client faced for the remaining nights.

Setting a Long-Range Daytime Goal

We set goals for the day because "having nothing to get up for" is often a key contributor to spending too much time in bed. One small step toward the goals for the day is then set for the coming week. Possible obstacles are identified and solved week by week.

Managing Low Energy and Fatigue during the Day

The behavioral experiments and surveys described in Chapter 4 are helpful for managing the decreased energy and fatigue experienced by many clients. For example, clients can benefit from completing an energy experiment in which they've learned that spending energy can be a useful way to generate energy. At other times, we can develop an experiment in which clients are asked to rate their mood and energy before and after engaging in a social activity or leaving the house to illustrate that contextual variables can improve mood and sleepiness. Creating a survey in which clients collect data on the strategies others use to generate energy, to get out of bed, or to fill in their time when they are bored is another helpful approach. Finally, remind the client that selective attention to salient internal threat cues (e.g., feelings of tiredness or fatigue) can cause him or her to worry or to change the plan for the day (Neitzert Semler & Harvey, 2004). Experiments on monitoring for fatigue and other signs of inadequate sleep (i.e., internal/bodily focus of attention) versus monitoring external stimuli can be helpful in breaking the tendency to be too vigilant about internal threat cues.

Optional Module 3: Dealing with Delayed or Advanced Phase

When to Use Optional Module 3

If bedtime is later or earlier than is preferred by the client, or is later than 2:00 A.M., or if midsleep times are outside of the 2:00 A.M. to 4:00 A.M. window over the course of 7 days of the sleep diary, we deliver Optional Module 3, starting around Session 4.

Background

Optimizing the timing of sleep is a core dimension of the sleep health frame-work. Problematic sleep timing can take the form of a delayed phase (late bed-times and late wake times) or an advanced phase (early bedtimes and early wake times). In the following section we provide some background related to delayed and advanced phase. Then we set forth treatment principles that can be adapted to address both problems.

As described in Chapter 2, the broader spectrum of eveningness is very common (Lovato et al., 2013), rather than the extreme end represented by the DSPT disorder. The full continuum is covered by this module. The approach adopted in TranS-C has been informed by the treatment literature on DSPT (Gradisar et al., 2011; Gradisar et al., 2014; Okawa et al., 1998; Regestein & Monk, 1995), as well as practice parameters (Sack et al., 2007). The overall goal is to assist the client in establishing strong habits of exposure to natural light in the morning and to dim light with electronic curfews in the evening.

Interventions

Rationale

For clients who have a tendency toward a delayed *phase*—i.e., bedtimes and wake times much later than desired—we provide the rationale for delivering this module by explaining that the human circadian system runs at approxi-mately 24 hours and 10 minutes. So unless we can resynchronize back to the 24-hour cycle, by the end of a week we will be 1 hour late for work and by the end of a month we will be 4 hours late. Evolution has endowed humans with the ability to naturally make use of specific environmental cues that help us entrain back to the 24-hour clock. In the sleep and circadian literature, these cues are referred to as *zeitgebers*, the German word for time givers. Light is the most powerful zeitgeber. Other powerful zeitgebers include regular mealtimes, exercise times, and social times. The *timing* of zeitgebers is also important. For instance, light *in the morning* advances sleep to an earlier time, but light *in the evening* delays sleep; and vice versa for darkness. This is why we recommend light in the morning and darkness in the evening. The handout associated with Cross-Cutting Module 2 (Appendix 4) can also be reviewed to facilitate the presentation of the rationale for this module.

Clients who have a tendency toward an *advanced phase*—i.e., bedtimes and waketimes much earlier than desired—often have few activities and lack social connections, which lead them to retire very early. This results either in clients lying in bed wide awake for hours as their body is simply not ready for sleep or in falling asleep and waking up very early if their circadian rhythm adjusts. Waking early in the morning can be distressing and frustrating because no one else is awake, and people often struggle to find something to do with their time. For these clients, it is important to explain that going to bed later actually means getting to sleep faster and at a preferred time. The circadian clock ensures that peak alertness and performance occurs in the day and a consolidated sleep period occurs at night. This rationale identifies the need to add daytime activities in order to delay bedtime and realign the circadian rhythm for peak daytime performance, better social engagement, and improved nighttime sleep. Activity planning includes consideration of meal times and activities between an evening meal and the initiation of the wind-down routine as described in Core Module 1, Part B. Once again the wind-down routine needs detailed planning on a practical level, for example, getting a new box set of a favorite TV series to watch or reading a book or magazine.

Advancing or Delaying Bedtime

When clients have a later or earlier bedtime than they prefer, work collaboratively to progressively move the bedtime earlier (for delayed phase) or later (for advanced phase) in 20–30 minute increments per week. The circadian system can tolerate larger shifts but, as described earlier, 20–30 minutes is a small enough shift for the system to adapt to and helps the client feel a sense of mastery. To support the adjustments to the sleep schedule, we review the importance of regular wake-up times *and* bedtimes, referring back to the client's sleep diary to check regularity and variability. We emphasize a regular morning wake-up time for delayed phase clients and a regular bedtime for advanced phase clients. We also note that the homeostatic sleep drive helps us to feel sleepy at night but can be discharged by late afternoon or evening naps.

Create a plan for how to achieve the bedtime and wake time goals, write the plan down, and then review strategies to enhance success. For example, (1) ask your client if he or she would like to consider setting an electronic curfew and an earlier or later bedtime (e.g., setting the client's cellphone alarm as a reminder of the time the wind-down should start); (2) suggest the client secure support from family and friends; (3) use an alarm clock to maintain a regular rising time; (4) brainstorm alternate strategies to daytime napping or caffeine use; and (5) emphasize key points about circadian rhythm with an emphasis on the advanced and delayed phases. For example, we can keep our biological clock in alignment by encouraging light exposure at around the same time each morning. Also, the SCN within the circadian system is the conductor of the orchestra of biological clocks—consistent bedtimes and rise times help keep the orchestra in tune. A key challenge for clients with delayed phase is waking up earlier in the morning, and for this group the RISE-UP routine (Core Module 1, Part C) is particularly beneficial. For clients with advanced phase, emphasize evening light and morning darkness.

Optional Module 4:
Reducing Sleep-Related Worry and Vigilance

When to Use Optional Module 4

The Anxiety and Preoccupation about Sleep Questionnaire (APSQ) is a 10-item self-report measure that assesses sleep-related worry (Tang & Harvey, 2004). The items are summed to obtain a total score that ranges from 10 to 100, with a higher score indicating more worry. If the client scores more than 60, we recommend administering Optional Module 4 typically starting around Session 5, although timing delivery early for clients who are experiencing worry at a level that impedes progress on the core modules is advisable.

Background

People with sleep problems often worry while trying to get to sleep at the beginning of the night, after waking in the middle of the night, on waking too early in the morning, and during the daytime. Anxiety is antithetical to sleep (Espie, 2002). Because excessive worry and rumination fuel anxiety and arousal, it is important to teach clients skills to manage unwanted thoughts.

Interventions

Revisiting the Wind-Down

Revisit the importance of the wind-down and consider adding strategies to specifically help disengaging from, and processing, the day. Examples of useful additions to the wind-down are described below.

Introducing Thinking Traps

Introduce "thinking traps" (see Appendix 11) from the classic work of Aaron T. Beck (1976). We emphasize that *everyone* falls into at least one of these traps. When you introduce each trap, try to illustrate it with examples that are relevant to the client and to sleep. As you continue, check each trap with the client to see if she or he recognizes it. Place a mark next to the traps your client recognizes. Ask for examples of each trap from the client's life. Sleep-related thinking traps are best, but if nonsleep traps are mentioned, go with them. For homework during the coming week, ask the client to monitor instances when he or she falls into a thinking trap, and for every time this happens, ask the client to add a mark next to the relevant trap. Check this homework the following week. If the client is prone to thinking traps, continue to check in on the process of the client catching himself or herself falling into thinking traps in each session and use the other interventions within this module—particularly the Negative Automatic Thoughts form—to teach the skills of how to evaluate their thinking traps. While we emphasize the relevance of thinking traps to sleep problems, we also believe that the skills for catching and evaluating thinking traps can be applied in many aspects of life.

Options for Managing Unwanted Thoughts

A menu of options for managing unwanted thoughts is shown in Box 5.2. Introduce each option, and then both client and therapist should practice each *in the session*. In-session practice is essential for ensuring that the client has a good understanding of the technique and affords an opportunity to troubleshoot and remove obstacles before the client tries the skill at home.

Why do we recommend that the therapist try the menu of options on his or her own worries at the same time as the client? This practice has a number of benefits, including the additional perspective that the therapist can bring to the experience. It also strengthens the alliance and the sense of collaboration between therapist and client. An entire session might be devoted to working through the menu items or, perhaps more effectively, introducing one or two strategies in every session.

Several of these strategies ask the client to focus on the positives in their life (e.g., savoring, practicing gratitude). An additional rationale for these approaches is that they have the potential to build rapid, automatic associative connections with a positive valence. For so many of us, the head hitting the pillow has become associated with worry and rumination. This menu of options is an opportunity to teach the client to reassociate sleep onset with positive valenced thought rather than with worry and rumination.

Look for opportunities to reinforce the essence of the cognitive model; namely, that thoughts trigger emotions. For example, the client might notice a mood change after trying some of the exercises in the session. This is an opportunity to point out that by changing our thinking (e.g., savoring rather than worrying), we can shift our mood.

BOX 5.2. Menu of Options to Manage the Mind

If you're feeling so anxious, stressed, or excited that you can't relax at night, try one of the following ways to manage worry and relax the mind. These skills can take time to master, so stick with them!

- **Practicing gratitude:** Try to generate three things that you are thankful for. Start with "I am grateful for. . . ."

- **Savoring:** Recall good feelings that you had today. What made you feel happy? Try to picture the situation and relive the feelings. Small things— like putting on a sweater and feeling warm on a cold day—are perfect for savoring.

- **Setting a "worry time" 2+ hours before bedtime:** Set aside a time to "worry"—that is, to think, write, and reflect about the important issues on your mind. Take your worry time at least 2 hours before bed so that your mind can fully relax by bedtime.

- **Problem solving:** Create two columns. Label one of the columns "Concerns" and the other column "Solutions." Then select a problem that you think might make it difficult to get to sleep. List this problem under "Concerns." Then, generate one next step that might contribute to solving this problem. Add it under "Solutions." Recognize that this is unlikely to be the final or full solution, as most problems have to be solved in steps. At least you have a first step in place!

- **Journaling**: You can have a special journal or just a blank sheet of paper for writing thoughts down in the evening. Anyone, anywhere, can journal. Writing down your thoughts and feelings can help clear your mind and relax you before sleep. You don't need to find solutions. It's all about the writing!

- **Using imagery:** Close your eyes and imagine a scene that is pleasant (e.g., a favorite holiday spot) but not overly arousing (e.g., not a car race). It needs to hold your attention and keep you relaxed at the same time. Ask yourself questions to engage all five senses: What do you SEE? What do you HEAR? What do you SMELL? What do you TASTE? What do you FEEL?

We emphasize that, as with any new skill, practicing over and over is necessary to form a habit. Perhaps end the practice by saying, "It is so great that you have derived benefit from this approach already. Given this, I encourage you to make this a habit, a bit like cleaning your teeth. But remember that it's hard to create new habits; it takes a lot of effort. What can you do to ensure you keep up the practice?" We encourage you to refer back to Cross-Cutting Module 3 for skills that promote habit formation. Remember to check the client's progress during every subsequent session.

Finally, most of these menu options have an evidence base for helping to reduce worry and rumination and/or improving sleep, including practicing gratitude (Wood, Joseph, Lloyd, & Atkins, 2009), savoring (McMakin, Siegle, & Shirk, 2011), constructive worry and problem solving (Carney & Waters, 2006), journaling (Harvey & Farrell, 2003), and imagery (Harvey & Payne, 2002).

Negative Automatic Thoughts

These offerings are relatively simple approaches and work well for many clients. However, when they are not sufficient, we should actually instruct the client in how to identify and evaluate worrisome, ruminative thoughts. The cognitive therapy texts by Aaron and Judith Beck are helpful for teaching these skills (A. T. Beck, 1979; J. S. Beck, 2005). Based on these approaches, here is a brief summary of the approach used in TranS-C.

INTRODUCING AND DEFINING AUTOMATIC THOUGHTS

We begin by defining negative automatic thoughts (NATs). The definition we use, drawn from A. T. Beck (1976), is presented in Box 5.3. If you think the client would understand the concept better using a different term, feel free to replace NATs with another term such as unhelpful thoughts, worry, or concerns. Give real-world examples to explain the concepts in Box 5.3. "As I am talking to you right now, I was also aware of the thought 'Oh, what's the time? I want to make sure we get through the agenda today.' So that's what is meant here on the handout (Box 5.3) by 'Train of thought that runs parallel with spoken thought.'" Then check in with the client as to whether he or she understands by asking: "Are you aware of this stream of thought too—the constant chatter running through our minds?" We emphasize that the mind is really never still, and that much of the content that runs through our minds is accepted as fact without an opportunity to logically evaluate it.

BOX 5.3. Automatic Thoughts

What Are Automatic Thoughts?

- They are a train of thought that runs parallel with spoken thought.
- We are often not fully aware of them.
- They typically emerge automatically and are extremely rapid.
- They sometimes occur in shorthand, a telegraphic style containing only the essential words.
- They do not arise as a result of deliberation, reasoning, or reflection; the thoughts just happen, like a reflex.
- They are often difficult to turn off.
- Usually the validity of the thoughts is accepted without question and without testing reality or logic.
- They often precede a powerful emotion.

We have hundreds and hundreds of negative automatic thoughts each day. The ones we are going to be particularly interested in are those that happen just before a strong emotion.

Ways to Manage Automatic Thoughts

This week:

- Observe them and report them. Two ways to observe them are (1) be attentive to the inner chatter and (2) when you notice a change in your emotions ask yourself, "What was going through my mind just before I started feeling this way?"

Next week we'll think about:

- Testing out the reality and logic of the thoughts and recognizing that they can be unreliable.

CATCHING AUTOMATIC THOUGHTS

Introduce the idea that it can be valuable to catch, spot, or become aware of automatic thoughts. To help with this process we introduce the Capturing Negative Automatic Thoughts form (see Appendix 14) and complete several examples in the session (see Box 5.4 for an example). Ideally the examples are drawn from the client's experiences over the last week and are related to sleep. If the client isn't able to recall specific thoughts, start with an emotion (e.g., feeling sad on waking) as the anchor and then work backward to uncover the thoughts that were driving the emotion. For homework, ask the client to monitor their NATs relating to the sleep problem (e.g., "I'm exhausted," "I am worried I won't get to sleep tonight"). Be sure to explain the rationale for this homework: "Once you get good at catching the thoughts, you'll be able to move on to working out what to do with them."

REVIEWING THE PREVIOUS WEEK'S
CAPTURING NEGATIVE AUTOMATIC THOUGHTS FORM

In the session that follows, we review the three-column NATs record form that was completed for homework. If it becomes apparent that the client hasn't understood the basic idea (e.g., they have "automatic thoughts" in the "emotions" column or vice versa), we discuss several more examples together. If you think the basic idea has been mastered (i.e., the client has successfully

---

BOX 5.4. Capturing Negative Automatic Thoughts Form

Situation	Emotion	Automatic Thoughts
When I woke up last Tuesday morning (7 A.M.)	Exhausted	Here we go again. I feel terrible. Wish I could sleep in. I can't cope.
At 2 A.M. last night	Anxious Uptight Angry	Oh no, it's 2 A.M. This is ruining my life. I've got to get back to sleep.

differentiated between "Situation," "Emotion," and "Automatic Thoughts"), move on to the next step (evaluating NATs). If not, consider asking the client to try the three-column form for 1 more week before moving on.

EVALUATING NATS

Using the Evaluating Negative Automatic Thoughts form (see Appendix 15), demonstrate the process of evaluating NATs. This will have the most impact if you evaluate a captured thought that is very "hot," or that is very meaningful to the client and contributes to distress. This thought might come from the Capturing Negative Automatic Thoughts form completed the previous week or, if the daily sleep diary indicated that the client had a particularly difficult night or a particularly difficult day in the past week, then ask about the thoughts that were experienced during that episode. Base the example on these thoughts. As always, make sure the thought you base the example on is sleep-related. The example of a completed form in Box 5.5 (also provided as a blank version in Appendix 15) is based on a format proposed by Judith Beck (2011). We selectively follow up and reinforce some of the answers the client gives to the questions on the form. Example follow-up questions are "That's really interesting—so thinking 'restate the thought' makes you feel anxious and you think is unhelpful for getting to sleep"; and "So that's interesting too—it seems you are finding more evidence for your hypothesis that the thoughts are affecting your sleep."

Key points to cover during this part of the module include the following.

- In very high emotion situations there will be lots of NATs. Encourage the client to write *all* of the thoughts down and then go back to circle the "hottest" thoughts. The hottest thoughts are the ones associated with the most emotion and distress. Complete the form based on these thoughts.

- Emphasize that when evaluating thoughts it is important to be absolutely honest, as opposed to trying to come up with an answer the client thinks will be acceptable or pleasing to you, their therapist.

- Use a negative emotion (e.g., anxiety) as a cue to look for, identify, and evaluate thoughts (some people tend to be more aware of the emotion than the thought).

- An emotion and an NAT are often in shorthand form. They can be easily unpacked by asking for the meaning of the thought.

- NATs may be in verbal form, images, or both.

BOX 5.5. Example of a Completed Evaluating Negative Automatic Thoughts Form

Negative Thought:
I bet I'm going to sleep badly tonight—this will be a disaster as we have my husband's parents coming over for lunch tomorrow.

Current Situation:
Saturday 9:30 P.M. Watching TV with husband (kids in bed).

Current Emotions:
Anxiety (90)

Evaluate Your Negative Thought

1. Is there an alternative way of thinking in this situation?
   I may be feeling anxious because I really want to impress my parents-in-law.

2. What is the evidence *for* my thought? What is the evidence *against* my thought?
   For—I have slept badly lately.
   Against—Even when I've slept badly, I feel OK the next day.

3. What's the worst that could happen? How likely is it? Could I live through it?
   I sleep badly and feel tired tomorrow. 60%. Yes. I could live through it.

4. What's the best that could happen? How likely is it? What's the most realistic outcome?
   I sleep fine and feel lively tomorrow. Seems 80% likely. I guess that's also the most realistic outcome, too.

5. What effect does thinking this thought have on me? Is my thought helpful?
   Will make it more likely to happen. No, these thoughts are not helpful.

6. What effect could changing my thought have on me?
   I'll be more likely to sleep well.

7. If a good friend was in this situation, what would I tell that friend?
   Chill out!

8. How important will this situation seem when I'm 80 years old?
   Not at all.

Outcome: What are you thinking and feeling now?
Anxiety (20)

- NATs can be evaluated for validity and for whether they are useful or helpful thoughts.

- Watch for themes. One client had many thoughts comparing the present to the past and often thought about how much better everything was in the past. These themes are often clues to core beliefs that can also be evaluated.

- Make the point that some NATs are unrealistic and need to be evaluated, whereas some NATs point to a need for a problem-solving approach. As a therapist it is important to teach the client how to differentiate between these two categories of thought: unrealistic thoughts that the Negative Automatic Thoughts form is useful for (e.g., "I can't cope with my work") and thoughts that require problem solving (e.g., "My husband is out of work, and we have severe financial problems").

After completing several examples together using the Evaluating Negative Automatic Thoughts form, give multiple copies of the blank form to the client to complete for homework over the coming week. Encourage the client to complete one form daily. The rationale is that it will take some time and practice to change thinking habits that have become ingrained over many years. Completing the form once or twice will not affect the habitual ways of thinking. The best way to develop a new style of thinking is by practice. Practice is also essential for breaking a habit!

In subsequent sessions, we check on how the client is managing with the new habit of spotting and evaluating his or her NATs. Review one or two more examples that the client completed for homework in each session to hone the skill. If this skill is practiced between and within sessions for several weeks, the client's thinking style will fundamentally change. For problems with this intervention we highly recommend Judith Beck's book (2005).

Introducing the Consequences of Thought Suppression

We also introduce the potential adverse consequences of thought suppression. For example, as soon as a client mentions strategies to cope with worry and rumination, such as "I try to suppress my thoughts" or "I try to clear my mind," we do the "white bear experiment" to illustrate the paradoxical effects of thought suppression (Harvey, 2016). The white bear experiment involves asking clients to find a comfortable seating position, and then to close their eyes. They spend several minutes trying to suppress all thought, particularly thoughts of a big, white, fluffy polar bear (or something your client likes—cars, football, cats, etc.). Do this thought exercise at the same time that your client tries it. After a few minutes, stop and discuss the result by asking, "How was that?" and "What do you conclude about the link between suppressing a thought and experiencing a thought?" We use these responses, and share our own experience, to educate the client about the paradoxical effects of thought suppression. This experiment is typically a compelling example of the adverse consequences of suppression. Here we interject that, in the spirit of the behavioral-experiment approach, wherever possible we set up an experience to demonstrate a point by *doing* rather than just *talking* about it—*doing* is a much more powerful platform for learning! Then we engage in a discussion about doing the opposite of suppression—letting the thoughts drift in and out. Part of the reason worry can feel so out of control is because of the "white bear effect" (Wegner, Schneider, Carter, & White, 1987). By removing suppression and letting thoughts come and go, the thoughts should have less strength and power. The strategies reviewed in Box 5.2 are also helpful alternatives to thought suppression.

Altering Problematic Beliefs about Sleep

Many clients hold beliefs about sleep that fuel worry and rumination. Examples include "If I don't get 8 hours of sleep every night, I won't be able to cope at work and I will lose my job" or "If I don't get to sleep soon, my health will start to suffer." For these clients, use Core Module 3, which focuses on altering unhelpful beliefs.

Discussing Positive Beliefs about Worry

A subgroup of clients hold beliefs about the benefits of worry, such as "Worrying in bed will help me get my mind straight" and "Worrying in bed will help me cope and prepare for the future." If the client has many positive beliefs about the utility of presleep worry, we discuss the pros and cons and consider doing behavioral experiments to collect data on whether the positive beliefs about worrying in bed are helpful or not.

Countering Vigilance and Monitoring for Sleep-Related Threat

Being vigilant and monitoring for sleep-related threat during the sleep onset period and during awakenings after sleep onset in the course of the night contribute to worry and rumination (Semler & Harvey, 2004). Consider the following examples.

While Colin was trying to fall asleep, he was always particularly alert to how close his body was to falling asleep. He would be on the lookout for the physical signs of drifting off, such as a slowing heart rate and a loss of muscle tone. When he detected these sensations, he'd think "Oh great, I'm finally falling asleep," which would pull him out of the delicious drifting off feeling and jerk him back to wakefulness, arousal, and anxiety about not being able to get to sleep.

Maryanne always turned out the light at 11:00 P.M. Then she would monitor her clock to see how long it was taking her to fall asleep. Every time she looked at the clock she'd think, "I hope I get to sleep soon." As the clock ticked on she'd start to think, "Oh no, this is terrible, I've *got* to get to sleep soon" and "If I don't get to sleep soon, I'm not going to cope tomorrow." These thoughts would cause Maryanne to feel anxious and aroused, making it even more difficult for her to fall asleep.

Immediately on waking Sally would monitor her body to see whether it was sufficiently rested. She nearly always noticed that her muscles felt sore and tired and that her eyes felt heavy. She'd then think, "Oh no! I didn't get enough sleep last night." This would make her feel sad and also anxious as she worried about how she would cope with the day ahead.

If such vigilance is present, we educate the client by sharing the Monitoring for Information about Sleep handout (see Box 5.6). The consequences of monitoring for the client can be profound. For example, one client monitored the sounds in his flat during the night. Over time they became so deafening that he had to move to a different flat. He came to treatment just as he was considering moving for the third time. Another client monitored feeling miserable all day and noticed that the miserable feelings increased. The situation is similar to that of monitoring a dripping faucet or a ticking clock and noticing that, the more you listen, the louder sounds of the dripping and ticking become.

Collaboratively devising behavioral experiments is a very effective way of working with monitoring behaviors. As evident from the examples below, vigilance and monitoring for sleep-related threat also occurs in the day. For example:

- Ask the client to monitor his or her legs for the next 5 minutes for itchy feelings. The client will find that paying attention to itchy feelings increases the need to scratch. This in-session behavioral experiment is borrowed from the treatment for panic disorder by Clark et al. (1999) and demonstrates that if we monitor for threat (e.g., feeling of fatigue while at work) these feelings can amplify.

BOX 5.6. Monitoring for Information about Sleep

While trying to get to sleep, do you monitor . . .

- Your body sensations for signs consistent with falling asleep (e.g., physical signs of drifting off, such as slowing heart rate, loss of muscle tone)?
- Your body sensations for signs inconsistent with falling asleep (e.g., heart pounding quickly, muscle tension)?
- The environment for signs of not falling asleep (e.g., noises outside and inside the house)?
- The clock to see how long it is taking you to fall asleep?
- The clock to calculate how much sleep will be obtained?

Waking in the morning, do you monitor . . .

- Your body sensations on waking for signs of poor sleep (e.g., heavy feeling in the head; heavy, tired eyes)?
- The clock on waking to calculate how many hours of sleep were obtained?

During the day, do you monitor . . .

- Your body sensations for signs of fatigue (e.g., heavy legs, sore shoulders)?
- Your performance for signs that attention, memory, or concentration is failing?
- Your mood for indications of tiredness or not coping?

- As also suggested in Core Module 2, go for a walk together in session time; both of you should spend 5 minutes internally monitoring how your body feels, paying particular attention to signs of tiredness and fatigue. Then rate how you feel. Then spend 5 minutes focusing externally on the trees, flowers, and sky, and rate how you feel. Go back to your office to debrief. Typically the switch in attentional focus externally has noticeable positive effects on energy levels, emotion, and worry.

• The essential feature of these between-session experiments (also in Core Module 2) is to give the client the experience of directing his or her attention outward, smelling the flowers, turning the radar off, and getting lost in the world around them. One possible way to do this involves a weekend hike in which the client spends 30 minutes asking questions like, 'How do my legs feel right now?' 'How does my torso feel right now?' and 'What about my shoulders and head, how do they feel?' Then the client rates (on a 0–10 scale, in a small notebook) the levels of tiredness and energy and the enjoyment of the walk. Then he or she spends 30 minutes asking questions like 'What can I see?' 'Is the scenery pleasant?' and 'Are the wildflowers out?' Then rerate the levels of tiredness and energy and enjoyment of the walk. Or ask the client to spend from 9:00 to 10:00 A.M. one morning monitoring how tired he or she is every 5 minutes, and then record how that feels. Then spend from 10:00 to 11:00 A.M. not monitoring at all, and record how that feels.

Other helpful points include:

• Explain that this ability to listen during sleep has evolutionary significance. For early humans, the ability to hear and respond to intruders during sleep, particularly large animals who were searching for food, was critical. New parents are particularly attuned to, and can easily hear, their newborn baby cry. In other words, noise that has particular relevance for our own or our loved ones' survival is going to easily arouse us from sleep.

• It is often helpful to use the metaphor of radar for vigilant monitoring during the night. One client had her radar on all night for the sound of the milk truck. Her alertness for the sound made it more difficult to get to sleep; she was easily woken by sounds similar to the milk truck, and when she finally woke up it was harder to get back to sleep because she was worried about not getting enough sleep and not coping the next day.

• Also, monitoring seems to increase when the client is bored. This is significant because a common safety behavior of clients who have not had enough sleep is to reduce their activity levels (e.g., skip aerobics or cancel plans for the day). Such safety behaviors allow more time and space to monitor, which then fuels arousal and worry.

As a way to summarize the findings of this module, ask the client to list his or her helpful and unhelpful strategies for managing worry (see Box 5.7 for an example). This list can be reviewed, extended, and updated as the sessions progress.

BOX 5.7. "Unhelpful" and "Helpful" Strategies
for Managing Worrying or Unwanted Thoughts
for a 53-Year-Old Female with Insomnia

Unhelpful	Helpful
• Listen to the radio: short circuits natural rhythm, might not always have one available, on waking head is ringing. • Suppress the thoughts (remember the white bear experiment). • Worry and ruminate. • Avoid thinking traps.	• Evaluate the thought using the Evaluating Negative Automatic Thoughts form. • Distract with interesting and engaging imagery. • Let the thoughts and images come and go. This is the opposite of suppression (I might find that I get bored of them and so they stop bothering me). • Keep a journal to promote emotional processing and resolution of worries and concerns (but in another room, before bedtime). • Get involved in or consumed by feeling snug and warm. • Make a "to-do" list before bedtime.

Unhelpful strategies are associated with the nonresolution of worries and can even make them worse.

Optional Module 5: Promoting Compliance with the CPAP Machine/Exposure Therapy for Claustrophobic Reactions

When to Use Optional Module 5

We screen for obstructive sleep apnea (OSA) with the eight-item STOP-Bang questionnaire (Farney et al., 2011), which was discussed in Chapter 2. We recommend referring individuals at high risk for OSA (indicated by the STOP-Bang) to a sleep specialist, who can conduct a full evaluation with an overnight sleep study. If the overnight study indicates the need for CPAP, we assess whether Optional Module 5 is needed to help the client adapt to using CPAP every night. The assessment is conducted with the CPAP Habit Index (Broström et al., 2014), which is a five-item assessment of adherence to CPAP and the longer and more detailed Attitudes toward CPAP Use Questionnaire (Stepnowsky et al., 2002). The latter questionnaire includes an assessment of self-efficacy (five items; e.g., "I am confident that I can use CPAP regularly"), outcome expectations (two items; e.g., "How important do you believe regular use of CPAP is for controlling your sleep apnea"), social support (nine items; e.g., "I have people in my life who will support me in using CPAP regularly"), and knowledge (12 items; e.g., "One of the main symptoms of sleep apnea is excessive daytime sleepiness"). We then peruse the survey of the client's responses to each item and responses on the subscales to determine if he or she would benefit from this module. Indications for delivering this module are responses that suggest that CPAP use has not yet been established as a habit as well as indications that the client has low self-efficacy, low outcome expectations, low social support, and inadequate knowledge about CPAP.

Background

During sleep, all of our muscles show reduced tone, including the muscles that keep our upper airway open. Breathing in creates negative pressure in our chest and airways, which tends to "suck in" the relaxed upper airway muscles during sleep. An apnea occurs when these upper airway muscles collapse from this negative pressure. CPAP therapy treats sleep apnea by preventing upper airway collapse during sleep. A CPAP device consists of a small air compressor connected to a flexible hose, which in turn is connected to a mask that fits over the individual's nose (and sometimes the mouth). When the machine is turned on and the mask is in place, the client is breathing pressurized air, which acts as a "splint" to keep the airway open. Some clients may be prescribed variants of CPAP, such as bilevel positive airway pressure (BiPAP), which automatically lowers the pressure during expiration, or autotitrating CPAP or APAP, which automatically adjusts the air pressure across the night. For simplicity, we use CPAP to refer to all variants of positive airway pressure therapy.

Although CPAP can be dramatically helpful to some clients with apnea, the therapy and its variants can be difficult to tolerate. If the client needs assistance adjusting to CPAP, we administer the approaches developed by several groups of experts in this field (Bartlett, 2011a, 2011b; Means & Edinger, 2011; O'Connor Christian & Aloia, 2011). There is ample empirical evidence supporting the effectiveness of these approaches (Aloia et al., 2001; Aloia et al., 2007; Aloia, Stanchina, Arnedt, Malhotra, & Millman, 2005; Means & Edinger, 2011; Richards, Bartlett, Wong, Malouff, & Grunstein, 2007).

Two problems are commonly encountered by clients as they adapt to CPAP.

1. A subgroup of clients don't use their CPAP for long enough during the night because they find the equipment uncomfortable. Most studies suggest that the benefits of CPAP on health and functioning require use for a minimum of 4 hours per night, although more is better. In these cases we use education on apnea (discussed in the next section) and the behavior-change approach described in Cross-Cutting module 3.

2. Another subgroup of clients experience claustrophobia when they use their CPAP. Claustrophobia is composed of two types of fears: fear of restriction and fear of suffocation. In these cases, we take a graded-exposure approach to help eliminate the link to anxiety and foster adherence to CPAP. We work toward the client viewing CPAP as safe and an investment in one's long-term health.

Interventions

Education on Apnea and CPAP

For both problems, education on sleep apnea and CPAP is a helpful starting point. First, we review the symptoms of sleep apnea and ask the client which symptoms they have experienced from the following list: loud snoring, breathing pauses, difficulty staying asleep, abrupt awakenings, and choking or gasping during sleep. Second, we review the daytime symptoms the client has experienced from the following list: excessive daytime sleepiness, fatigue, awakening with dry mouth, sore throat, chest pain, morning headache, difficulty concentrating, mood changes, and high blood pressure. Finally, we review the components of CPAP, which include the mask that fits over the nose and mouth, the straps that keep the mask in place, the tube that connects the mask to the machine's motor, and the motor that blows air into the tube.

Pros and Cons of Motivational Interviewing

Developed by Mark Aloia and colleagues (Aloia, Arnedt, Riggs, Hecht, & Borrelli, 2004), for clients who are underutilizing their CPAP, we use the responses to the Attitudes toward CPAP Use Questionnaire (Stepnowsky et al., 2002) to assess the client's readiness for and confidence about using CPAP, exploring ambivalence by reviewing the pros and cons of use and nonuse. On the pros side, clients are often aware of the health benefits. However, on the cons side, clients are often concerned about the CPAP causing them physical discomfort or claustrophobia or their appearance when wearing the mask. The therapist helps the client to identify consequences of use of CPAP that are particularly important to the client, including eliminating or greatly reducing the risk of heart disease, stroke, or hypertension. Any level of successful use is reinforced, and the therapist empathizes with the difficulties and the obstacles encountered. Then small goals are collaboratively derived that will promote the use of CPAP.

Assessing Claustrophobic Reactions

For clients who are experiencing claustrophobia, we explain that claustrophobic reactions to CPAP are common and that the problem is treatable. We start by assessing the scope of the problem by asking, "What is your experience using CPAP so far?" and "Do you experience this feeling in other situations?"

We review the purpose of the treatment, namely, to become comfortable with using CPAP and to promote adaptation to CPAP gradually through small steps and continual practice. We also review the rationale for exposure therapy, explaining that this involves (1) confronting the feared object or situation with help and support from a therapist, (2) learning to tolerate and manage fear without the need to escape or avoid the object/situation, and (3) increasing control over fear.

Exposure

We focus on helping the client to become more comfortable with CPAP while they are awake so that they can learn how to sleep easily with CPAP. We begin with an in-session exposure demonstration (shown in Step 1) and ask clients to complete between-session exposure for homework (shown in Steps 1–4). The graded exposure involves the following steps:

1. Switch the CPAP airflow to the on position. We ask the client to place the mask over his or her nose and breathe. Keep the mouth closed. Start with a short stint of a few minutes. Build up to longer periods of breathing over time.
2. Repeat Step 1, but this time ask the client to place the straps over his/her head too. The client should work his or her way up to wearing the mask comfortably for 15–20 minutes.
3. Ask the client to try taking a nap during the day with the mask on and the CPAP machine turned on. There is no pressure to fall off to sleep. Instead, the client should practice resting comfortably.
4. Have the client wear CPAP at night when going to sleep.

At any point, if the client experiences uncomfortable feelings, we suggest that he or she repeat the previous step to gain mastery before moving to next one.

In future sessions we assess adherence to homework, monitor progress via client self-report and objective CPAP data (many CPAP machines have inbuilt adherence monitors), and problem-solve obstacles. At times we conduct further in-session exposure trials.

Optional Module 6: Negotiating Sleep in a Complicated Environment

When to Use Optional Module 6

Deliver this module if there are environmental factors interfering with sleep. Home visits allow for the direct assessment of the sleep environment and enable the clinician to offer practical support to facilitate changes. We establish a safety plan for the home visit, and we consider possible liability issues prior to the visit. Another means of achieving a good assessment of the sleeping environment is to ask the client to take photographs of their home.

Background

Many environmental factors may interfere with the ability to sleep. Examples include not having a comfortable bed, homelessness, traffic noise, street light entering the bedroom, or pets who jump on and off the bed during the night (Waite et al., 2015). Working toward minimizing the impact of these issues is an important part of TranS-C.

Interventions

Solution Focus

We follow the approach of Daniel Freeman, Felicity Waite, and colleagues (Waite et al., 2015), which is practical and solution focused. When working toward deriving a solution to an environmental issue that is interfering with sleep, we set small and realistic goals that are important to the client. We ensure we are working toward goals that are positive, rather than negative (de Shazer & Dolan, 2012; Lloyd, 2008). For example, if the client decides to move the TV out of the bedroom, provide an intervention that replaces the function the television was serving. More specifically, if watching TV was a way to distract the client from worry and rumination, offer the skills from Optional Module 4.

The solution-focused approach also involves understanding that problems are maintained by doing more of the same. It assumes that clients have resources and strengths to resolve complaints. The emphasis is on acknowledging distress, focusing the conversation on success, and discussing solutions rather than problems. We concentrate on what is possible and changeable, rather than on what is impossible and intractable (de Shazer & Dolan, 2012; Lloyd, 2008).

Problem Solving

We also draw on the evidence-based problem-solving module from cognitive behavioral social skills training (CBSST; Granholm et al., 2013), which involves teaching the client the SCALE acronym: **S**pecify the problem, **C**onsider all possible solutions, **A**ssess the best solution, **L**ay out a plan, and **E**xecute and **E**valuate the outcome as an approach to solving problems.

Communication Skills

At times the sleep environment is shared, either with a partner or a roommate. In these situations it is often necessary to teach the client communication skills to calmly but assertively facilitate establishing a quiet, calm, safe, and positive space for sleep. Again, we borrow content from CBSST (Granholm et al., 2013). The predominant approach is to role play problem solving with roommates. The client is encouraged to practice expressing positive and negative feelings, with the emphasis on making a positive request. After each role play, the client thinks through the strengths and weaknesses of the approach taken. Thoughts and beliefs (e.g., "nothing will ever change") are assessed, as they often present barriers to successful communication.

Finances

It is important to be sensitive to the financial resources of each client. For example, if a client has been homeless and has just found a bed in a group home, it is usually not helpful to point out the problems with the group-home environment and suggest that the client find another place to live. This can be destabilizing at a critical time, and is insensitive to how hard it can be for homeless people to find decent accommodations. Having a bed to sleep in (even if not ideal) is better than having no bed at all. Also, it may not be possible for the client to buy a new, more comfortable mattress or blinds to darken the bedroom. Thus, we try working with the client to find creative ways to modify his or her sleeping environment, such as using towels or a tablecloth to block light coming into the window in the morning.

Optional Module 7: Reducing Nightmares

When to Use Optional Module 7

If the client reports having nightmares, add questions to the sleep diary that provide ongoing monitoring of the frequency, intensity, and disruptive aspect of nightmares, encouraging the client also to note the theme of the nightmare and the extent to which they are distressing. Often monitoring reveals that the nightmares are very rare, and therefore don't warrant spending session time on them. However, we offer this optional module, with the client's consent, when the frequency and intensity of nightmares are causing the client distress.

Background

Nightmares arise during REM sleep, typically in the second half of the night; this contrasts with sleepwalking and sleep terrors, which arise from deep non-REM sleep in the first half of the night. Nightmares are disturbing because the content of the dream or the emotions in the dream are unpleasant, and these features persist after the sleeper awakens. Seventy-five to 90% of people who experience stressful life events report nightmares.

Interventions

This module is based on research by Barry Krakow, Anne Germain, and their colleagues (Germain et al., 2007; Krakow et al., 2001). The evidence base for this approach to nightmares, imagery rehearsal therapy, is strong. Indeed, the therapy results in a significant reduction in the number of nightmares per week and in improved sleep. Interestingly, imagery rehearsal therapy has also been associated with a decrease in PTSD symptoms (Casement & Swanson, 2012).

Monitoring

The approach begins by adding several questions to the daily sleep diary to assess the frequency of the nightmares and the extent of the disruption they cause. Specifically, each night we ask the client to record (1) the number of dreams he or she remembers, (2) the number of nightmares he or she were aware of, and (3) the amount of distress experienced with each nightmare on a scale from 0 ("no distress") to 10 ("extreme distress"). We ask further questions to assess the impact of nightmares on the client's sleep and daytime functioning.

Imagery Rehearsal

The treatment phase begins by teaching the client how to use imagery rehearsal therapy on a single self-selected nightmare. We don't start with the most distressing nightmare, but rather with a nightmare that causes moderate distress (i.e., a significant but not overwhelming nightmare). The following steps are used:

1. Write down the dream.
2. Think of a way to change the dream in any way the client wishes.
3. Write down the modified dream.
4. Rehearse the modified dream using imagery for 3–5 minutes, always using the first person and the present tense. The client is invited to close his or her eyes if they are comfortable. If the client prefers, an alternative is to find a point on the floor on which to fixate. We also assist the client in forming mental images of the dream, rather than just using verbal thought to go through the dream.
5. We assess how the imagery session and the new dream feels and if some modification is needed.

We complete these steps together in the session. Then, for homework, we ask the client to spend time each day practicing imagery rehearsal. The recommendation is to rehearse no more than two new dreams each week. We reassure the client that practice makes perfect; the more the new dream images are repeated, the better he or she will be able to replace bad dreams.

Conclusions and Future Directions

We commenced this book by introducing the sleep health framework that underlies TranS-C. We emphasized that TranS-C, and all interventions for sleep and circadian problems, should not stop at treating sleep and circadian disorders and dysfunction, although this is an important goal. The sleep health framework encourages us to go much further and pursue the larger goal of *promoting sleep health* across multiple empirically derived domains.

In Chapter 1, we reviewed the evidence linking aspects of sleep with mental and physical health outcomes. Based on this evidence, a successful course of treatment is defined by measurable improvement along the following six sleep health dimensions: the client is more *satisfied* with his or her sleep or sleep quality; the client is more *alert* during waking hours and is less sleepy in the daytime; the *timing* of the client's sleep within the 24-hour day is during the nighttime hours of darkness; the client's sleep is *efficient* in that the relative amount of time spent in bed is similar to the time spent asleep; the total *duration* of sleep obtained per 24 hours is appropriate given the age of the client; and the client has developed the ability to go to sleep at *regular* times each night and wake at *regular* times each day. We proposed the four cross-cutting modules, four core modules, and the seven optional modules that comprise TranS-C to comprehensively promote improvement across the six sleep health dimensions.

The transdiagnostic potential of treating sleep and circadian problems is an exciting one. The approach allows treatment providers to address a broad range of common sleep problems that are associated with a broad range of mental and physical disorders. As such, TranS-C is designed to address the complexity of real-life sleep problems. Also, by producing one transdiagnostic protocol rather than multiple disorder-focused protocols, we hope this approach will help to address the "too many empirically supported treatments problem" noted by Weisz et al. (2014, p. 68).

In certain ways, the development of TranS-C is in its early days. While the elements that comprise TranS-C are empirically derived and are drawn from existing evidence-based treatments, there is a need for a large-scale evaluation of the approach. Thus far, one small randomized controlled trial has been conducted with individuals diagnosed with bipolar disorder, and two relatively large-scale randomized controlled trials, one for youth and one for adults, are in progress. The latter two trials are truly transdiagnostic in that the participants have a wide range of diagnoses and sleep and circadian problems, whereas the former trial is only transdiagnostic in that the individuals share a wide range of sleep and circadian problems. The data for the small adult study (Harvey et al., 2015) and the youth study indicate that TranS-C improves important aspects of sleep and circadian functioning and improves symptoms of comorbid problems. We await the results of the 6- and 12-month follow-up for the youth study, and initial results from the adult study will be available late in 2018.

An important next step is for further evaluations to be conducted by independent research groups, as this is one of the criteria required before declaring that a treatment has a "strong" evidence base (Chambless & Hollon, 1998) (www.psychologicaltreatments.org). In addition, research is needed to understand which clients TranS-C works best for and under which conditions. There also will be a need to identify and remove barriers at the client, therapist, organization, and government levels to the scaling of TranS-C to ensure that the current 15- to 20-year lag between the development of a treatment and its clinical availability (if it ever becomes available) is substantially reduced (Sorensen, Rawson, Guydish, & Zweben, 2003; Sundararaman, 2009).

There are a relatively small number of mental health professionals and they are concentrated in highly populated, affluent urban areas. Yet there is a wide geographical distribution of the people who desperately need treatment (Kazdin & Blase, 2011; Kazdin & Rabbitt, 2013). As such, there have been urgent calls to develop more 'spoons' (Yates, 2011) for delivering treatments like TranS-C to a more diverse group of clients via the Internet, telephone, smartphone, self-help book, text message, TV, radio (Kazdin & Blase, 2011), interactive computer programs, apps (Andersson, 2009; Teachman, 2014) and, in some circumstances, via home visits. Scaling would certainly be facilitated if TranS-C could be simplified still further so that nontraditional service providers could deliver the treatment (Kazdin & Blase, 2011; Kazdin & Rabbitt, 2013).

TranS-C also might be further enhanced by adding modules to address other factors that impact sleep. Prime candidates are food consumption and exercise. This trio of behaviors—diet, activity, and sleep—are major behavioral health risk factors, all of which are regulated by, and in turn influence, the circadian timing system. The circadian timing system serves as a unifying theme that underpins these major challenges to public health.

More specifically, we know that one night of poor sleep results in an increased intake of carbohydrates and fat, reduced protein intake, and increased caloric intake overall the following day (Brondel, Romer, Nougues, Touyarou, & Davenne, 2010). Consistently, Greer, Goldstein, and Walker (2013) reported that the desire for weight-gain-promoting foods increased after sleep deprivation in adults and was predicted by subjective daytime sleepiness. Moreover, excess weight and obesity are strongly associated with, and predict the onset of, sleep problems such as sleep apnea (Drager, Togeiro, Polotsky, & Lorenzi-Filho, 2013; Patel & Hu, 2008). There is evidence that sleep deprivation reduces physical activity and that increasing physical activity improves sleep (Chennaoui, Arnal, Sauvet, & Léger, 2015; Kline, 2014). Given the likely bidirectional causal pathways between sleep and exercise and sleep, food choice, and excess weight gain, more consideration should be given to addressing exercise and diet within TranS-C.

Given the very high rates of comorbidity among mental illnesses, a key challenge will be how to sequence or interweave treatment approaches for comorbid conditions. For example, when a client has both insomnia and depression, one choice is to sequence the treatments by providing the evidence-based treatment for depression first and then deliver the evidence-based treatment for insomnia. However, in light of the mounting evidence that mental illness and sleep problems are mutually maintaining (Harvey, 2008), an interwoven treatment may represent a significant advance over the sequential approach. A study conducted in collaboration with Greg Clarke from Kaiser Permanente, Oregon, in which we delivered CBT for depression and insomnia each week for youth has provided a preliminary evidence base for interwoven treatment. The treatment elements designed to target depression and the treatments designed to target insomnia were interwoven across the sessions, such that progress on each problem was made in most sessions. The results were very encouraging, in that specific insomnia and depression outcomes were in the medium-to-large effect size range (Clarke et al., 2015). We propose TranS-C as a prime candidate for interweaving with other evidence-based treatments, yet the specific details and guidelines for the interweaving approach are a topic for future work.

Given the huge need globally to improve sleep health, along with the scarcity of treatment providers who have the skills to deliver the help that is needed, we offer TranS-C as a simple, scalable, flexible, and hopefully powerful treatment for moving the field forward.

Appendices

Resources

Resources to Improve Motivation

The following articles can be incorporated into sessions based on the clients' interests. Each article addresses the importance of increasing sleep and/or modifying technology use in order to improve performance and health.

Sports

"While You Weren't Sleeping" (ESPN)
   http://espn.go.com/blog/truehoop/post/_/id/66479/while-you-werent-sleeping

"The Doctor Who Coaches Athletes on Sleep" (The Atlantic)
   www.theatlantic.com/health/archive/2014/04/for-better-performance-athletes-need-
      sleep/361042

"How to Sleep Your Way to a Sixpack" (WellnessFX)
   http://blog.wellnessfx.com/2014/10/09/ben-greenfield-sleep-six-pack

"Why Athletes Should Make Sleep a Priority in Their Daily Training" (Fatigue Science)
   www.fatiguescience.com/blog/infographic-why-athletes-should-make-sleep-a-priority-
      in-their-daily-training

"Sleep Is a Weapon" (Globe and Mail)
   www.theglobeandmail.com/sports/give-it-a-rest-sports-teams-learn-how-to-use-sleep-
      as-a-weapon/article21417789/?page=1

School Performance

"Want to Ace that Test? Get the Right Kind of Sleep" (New York Times)
   http://parenting.blogs.nytimes.com//2014/10/16/want-to-ace-that-test-get-the-right-kind-
      of-sleep

"Poor Sleep Tied to Kids' Lower Academic Performance" (Reuters)
   www.reuters.com/article/2013/08/16/us-health-poor-sleep-idUSBRE97F0UA20130816

"Multitasking Doesn't Just Hurt Productivity—It Could Damage Your Brain" (Business
   Insider)
   www.businessinsider.com/multitasking-could-damage-your-brain-2014-10

Health and Appearance

"Here's a Horrifying Picture of What Sleep Loss Will Do to You" (Huffington Post)
   www.huffingtonpost.com/2014/01/08/sleep-deprivation_n_4557142.html?utm_hp_
      ref=infographics

(continued)

"So What If You Don't Get Enough Sleep?" (Fast Company)
www.fastcodesign.com/1663126/infographic-of-the-day-so-what-if-you-dont-sleep-enough

"Hard Lesson in Sleep for Teenagers" (New York Times)
http://well.blogs.nytimes.com/2014/10/20/sleep-for-teenagers

"Want to Lose Weight? Kick These 'Friends' Out of Bed" (Huffington Post)
www.huffingtonpost.com/kellyann-petrucci/phones-sleep_b_5948604.html?&ncid=tweetlnkushpmg00000067

"Smartphones Ruin More Than Your Sleep" (Business Insider)
www.businessinsider.com/smartphones-effect-on-vision-and-health-2014-9

RISE-UP Humorous Approaches

Here are some creative options for new alarm clocks that promote a sense of humor when working on the RISE-UP routine.

https://youtu.be/izWCU4Y61o4 (Clocky)

http://mashable.com/2013/09/12/wake-n-shake-alarm-app

http://mashable.com/2011/08/17/iphone-alarm-clock-donates-your-snooze-to-charity

http://mashable.com/2011/05/29/money-shredding-alarm

Videos to Bring Sleep Concepts to Life

The following resources can be incorporated into sessions to engage clients and help the sleep concepts "stick."

To help explain the science of sleep:
https://youtu.be/pwNMvUXTgDY

To help explain the forces that control sleep and waking (homeostat and circadian):
http://healthysleep.med.harvard.edu/interactive/sleep-forces

To help explain the impact of jet lag:
https://youtu.be/ooUA0KF2FzM
https://youtu.be/7Mgg1mSg5C4
(All are videos of jet-lagged babies falling asleep while eating.)

To help explain what happens at daylight saving time:
www.psychologytoday.com/blog/chronotherapy/201403/escape-the-burden-switching-daylight-saving-time

To help explain why snoozing is a bad idea:
http://mashable.com/2013/03/21/the-science-of-snoozing

To help explain how social ties affect sleep:
http://mashable.com/2013/12/25/teen-sleep

To help explain how the teen brain works (for parents):
www.livescience.com/13850-10-facts-parent-teen-brain.html

A humorous approach to the RISE-UP routine:
www.youtube.com/watch?v=wDx7wrkhstg

To help explain maladaptive conditioning between the bed and sleep-incompatible activities:
www.youtube.com/watch?v=9RS-9m3dkg4

To build motivation for getting out of bed (for athletically inclined clients):
"Rise and Swim"
http://truthseekerdaily.com/2013/11/if-you-love-hitting-your-snooze-button-you-will-want-to-see-this-video

Personalized Case Conceptualization Form

	Things I do	Things I think	Things I feel
At bedtime			
Consequence:			
In the night			
Consequence:			
On waking			
Consequence:			
During the day			
Consequence:			

From *Treating Sleep Problems: A Transdiagnostic Approach* by Allison G. Harvey and Daniel J. Buysse. Copyright © 2018 The Guilford Press. Permission to photocopy this material is granted to purchasers of this book for personal use or use with individual clients (see copyright page for details). Purchasers can download enlarged versions of this material (see the box at the end of the table of contents).

APPENDIX 4

Understanding Sleep and What It Does for Us: Adults

A Rhythmic World

We live in a rhythmic world. The evidence is all around us.

- Night follows day.
- There are four seasons.
- Stars have annual patterns.
- Some flowers close at night and open during the day.
- Some birds migrate annually or biannually.

Body Rhythms

Like the physical world, our bodies have rhythms. These rhythms are built-in, or "endogenous." In other words, our rhythms are part of the normal function of our genes, cells, and organs. Our body rhythms are usually synchronized with the rhythms of the world, but staying synchronized requires good sleep and waking habits. There are actually several different types of body rhythms:

- Circadian @ 24 hours (e.g., sleep–wake rhythms)
- Ultradian < 24 hours (e.g., breathing and heart rhythms)
- Infradian > 24 hours (e.g., menstrual cycles)

Human Sleep

Sleep is the process through which our brains and bodies restore their efficient functioning. Contrary to common belief, sleep is not just the absence of wakefulness. It is an active process that has its own distinctive characteristics and structure.

- Sleeping is a period of rhythmic and substantial brain and body activity.
- On falling to sleep there is a rapid descent from lighter stages of sleep, called non-rapid-eye-movement (non-REM) Stages 1 and 2 (N1 and N2) to the deepest stages of sleep, called non-REM 3 (N3).
- Stage N3 is difficult to wake from. When you do awaken from N3, you may feel disoriented or confused.
- Stage N3 is important for:
  o Growth and repair and immune system functioning
  o Helping to retain long-term information and memories
  o Balancing out the body's hormones that make you hungry and affect your weight
- Stage N2 sleep is a lighter stage of sleep that:
  o Prepares the brain for next-day learning
  o Helps to build and maintain muscle memory, involved in playing sports or other physical activities
  o Helps us integrate new information into existing memories

(continued)

Note. Based on Carskadan and Dement (2017).

- REM or rapid-eye-movement sleep is a relatively active stage of sleep when most of our dreaming occurs. REM is important for:
  - Memory consolidation
  - Emotional processing
  - Creativity
- Non-REM and REM sleep are organized into 90- to 110-minute cycles across the night.
- We have more Stage N3 sleep in the first cycle, less in the second cycle, and small amounts in the third or fourth cycles. Also, there is a greater predominance of REM and non-REM Stage N2 sleep in the second half of the night.
- We get lighter stages of sleep (Stage N1, N2, and REM) in the morning. They are all fairly easy to wake up from.

Two Processes

Sleep is not a voluntary process. In other words, we can't just decide to sleep whenever we'd like. Rather, sleep is controlled by a number of factors, two of which are particularly important when thinking about normal sleep and sleep problems.

The two processes that control sleep are:

1. Homeostatic sleep drive: This is like "sleep pressure" that builds up with progressive wakefulness. The longer you're awake, the sleepier you get.
2. Circadian rhythm: It's not a coincidence that most people sleep at night and are awake during the day. We have a 24-hour (circadian) rhythm of sleep and wakefulness. The peak time of sleepiness for most people is between approximately 3:00 A.M. and 5:00 A.M.

These two processes work together in a good sleeper. We build up our homeostatic sleep drive throughout the day, which helps us to fall asleep at night. In the middle of the night, our circadian rhythms keep us asleep. We then wake up with a low homeostatic sleep drive and a rising circadian alertness rhythm.

These processes underlie important behavioral recommendations for better sleep.

- Stay awake long enough to get sleepy (homeostatic sleep drive).
- Keep your time in bed similar to the amount of time you can actually sleep (homeostatic drive).
- Sleep at night whenever possible (circadian rhythm).
- Keep to a regular sleep–wake schedule (circadian rhythm).

Melatonin

Melatonin is the "hormone of darkness." It follows a strong circadian rhythm, and is released only at night. Melatonin provides an internal signal of darkness and tells our brain to do what it should be doing at night (i.e., sleep).

- Released by the pineal gland.
- Helps us to feel sleepy.
- The pineal gland releases melatonin only if it's dark. Light at night suppresses melatonin.

(continued)

- Melatonin can be released only at night. It can't be released during the day even if it is dark!
- That means we can be awake way past a reasonable time if we are in the light, and our melatonin cannot kick in to help us fall asleep.

Light and Dark

Periods of light and dark at the right times are the most important signals to our biological clock. We need light at the same time each morning to help set our biological clock.

On the other hand, the following technologies at night are associated with light at the wrong time of day. These tell the brain that it is time to be awake, and do not promote sleepiness; instead they keep you up (not just because they are engaging, but also because they emit light!):

- TV
- Cellphones
- Text messages
- Internet/Facebook/Twitter

A Temporal Orchestra

- Every cell in your body has a biological clock and a rhythm.
- Your brain is like a conductor: It has the challenge of keeping tens of thousands of different clocks in your body synchronized!
- To keep your body's orchestra in sync, it is best to wake up around the same time each morning and go to bed around the same time each night and to follow as much of a daily rhythm as possible in all of our activities.

The Life-Changing Benefits of Consistency

To keep your orchestra of clocks in tune, it is best to wake up around the same time each morning and go to bed around the same time each night. Changing around your sleep–wake schedule has the same impact on you as traveling across time zones. It's also a good idea to keep activities like mealtimes, work, and exercising at consistent times. Keeping regular schedules helps the biological clock to do its job.

What time do you . . .

- Go to bed on weekdays?
- Wake up on weekdays?
- Go to bed on weekends?
- Wake up on weekends?

Are you chronically "jet-lagged"? To our biological clock, very irregular sleep–wake timing is almost equivalent to traveling across time zones.

149

Understanding Sleep and What It Does for Us: Youth

What Is Sleep?

Sleep is a periodic and reversible *state* during which the brain and body function differently than they do during wakefulness. Differences between sleep and wakefulness can be observed in a person's behavior, but they are also indicated by changes in the physiological activities of the brain and body. Sleep is characterized by a reduced awareness of, responsiveness to, and interaction with the environment. Sleep in humans is usually accompanied by lying down, low physical activity, and closed eyes.

Do you know the recommended amount of sleep for someone your age?
- Brain and body: 9 hours!
- Range: 8–10 hours

What's happening when we sleep?
- **Rapid-eye-movement (REM) sleep:** This is the stage of sleep during which most of our dreams occur. It is characterized by a paralysis of most of our muscles, but an active brain. Memory consolidation and emotional processing occur during REM.
- **Non-rapid-eye-movement (non-REM) Stage 1 (N1):** Light sleep. N1 can be thought of as a transitional state or a "bridge" between wakefulness and sleep. Some people feel that they are still awake during N1 sleep.
- **Non-REM Stage 2 (N2):** Medium-depth sleep, which takes up the most time during the night. Preparation for next-day learning is a key function of N2.
- **Non-REM Stage 3 (N3):** Deep sleep. Growth and repair of our bodies occurs during N3. This stage is also important for strengthening learning and memories. It occurs mostly in the first half of the night and is very difficult to awaken from.

Circadian Rhythms

- Circadian rhythms are equal to about a day, but slightly longer.
- Circadian rhythms help determine sleep patterns—when we feel sleepy and when we feel awake.
- Every morning, we entrain, or resync, with the 24-hour day outside.
- We entrain with the help of time cues:
  - Light
  - Social activities
  - Physical activity
  - Meals
  - Temperature

(continued)

Note. Based on Carskadon and Dement (2017).

A Temporal Orchestra

- Every cell in your body has a biological clock and a rhythm.
- Your brain is like an orchestra conductor: It has the challenge of keeping these rhythms synchronized!
- To keep your body's orchestra in sync, it is best to wake up around the same time each morning and go to bed around the same time each night and to follow as much of a daily rhythm as possible in all of our activities.

Crazy Sleep Schedules

To keep your orchestra of clocks in tune, it is best to wake up around the same time each morning and go to bed around the same time each night. Changing around your sleep–wake schedule has the same impact on you as traveling across time zones. It's also a good idea to keep activities like eating, working, and exercising at consistent times. Keeping regular schedules helps the biological clock do its job.

What time do you . . .

- Go to bed on weekdays?
- Wake up on weekdays?
- Go to bed on weekends?
- Wake up on weekends?

Are you chronically "jet-lagged"? If you go to bed or wake up more than 3 hours later on 1 day compared to the previous day, that's the equivalent (to your biological clock) of flying from Los Angeles to New York!

Melatonin

- Secreted by the pineal gland.
- Secreted only at night and only if it's dark.
- Inhibited by light.
- Helps us feel sleepy at the right time of day.

Light

- Interrupts production of melatonin.
- Even moderately bright light at night reduces melatonin.
- Directly increases alertness.
- Interferes with winding down toward sleepiness.

(continued)

151

Darkness

- A powerful cue for the biological clock.
- Triggers a cascade of biological processes that will help you fall asleep.

Do <u>not</u> turn on bright lights if you get up in the night (e.g., to use the restroom). Keep the lights as low as possible.

Nighttime Screen Time

Screen time is equal to light time, and light at night throws off our circadian rhythms. For the best sleep, keep all lights low at night, and avoid them when possible. That means 30–60 minutes prior to sleep, avoid:

- TV
- Gaming
- Texting
- Internet and social media (Instagram, Snapchat, Facebook, Kik, etc.)

Why Do You Use Tech at Night?

- Rewarding and fun?
- Time away from parents?
- FOMO ("fear of missing out")?
- Fear of being alone?
- Fear of bullying or exclusion if disconnected?

Form to Guide
Implementation Intentions and Mental Contrasting

This worksheet is likely to be very helpful because it is based on the growing science of achieving goals and changing habits so as to improve our lives. The techniques are known as mental contrasting (developed by Gabrielle Oettingen and her colleagues) and implementation intention (developed by Peter Gollwitzer and his colleagues).

Anticipated situation:

Goal:

What is it that would make it so good for you personally to seize your goal?

Let's spend a few minutes imagining your response as vividly as possible. Let yourself indulge in fantasizing about this positive outcome without considering the obstacles in the present reality.

What is the most critical obstacle that stands in the way of your seizing your goal?

(continued)

Let's spend a few minutes imagining the most critical obstacle as vividly as possible.

Does your goal involve a single action or a sequence of actions? Write down the single action or the sequence. For each action choose a specific point in time and a specific place when you will enact each action.

Action	Place	Time

Say out loud to yourself your commitment to seizing this goal. Use a form like:

"If/when I encounter this situation _____,

I intend to _____ **at this time** _____

in this _____ **place."**

Write down your commitment and then visualize it as vividly as possible.

Repeat it a few times. This is important.

My Sleep Goals

Choose goals that are specific and easy to track. Avoid choosing vague goals like "Get more sleep" and "Feel rested in the morning." Instead, choose specific goals like "Get into bed by [time] every night," "Turn off my phone and computer at [time]," and "Get 10 minutes of physical activity within 30 minutes of waking up in the morning."

Goals for Nighttime

1.

2.

3.

4.

Goals for Daytime

1.

2.

3.

4.

Once you've set your goals for nighttime and daytime, consider adding them as additional rows on your sleep diary so you can track your progress from week to week!

Winding Down at Night

What Is a Wind-Down Routine and Why Is It Important?

A wind-down routine is a set of behaviors—things you can do—to prepare your brain and body for sleep. Remember that sleep is not a voluntary process. In other words, you can't simply decide that you are going to sleep and make it happen. Rather, sleep occurs when our brain and body are ready for it, based on how long we have been awake, the time of day (or night), and what is going on at the moment. A wind-down routine focuses on the last factor—what is going on at the moment—and makes sure that you have the best circumstances for allowing sleep to happen.

Questions

- What time do you typically go to bed?
- Is there a range of times throughout the week? If so, why?
- Do you do anything particular to get ready for bed? If so, what do you do?
- How alert or sleepy do you feel at bedtime?

Suprachiasmatic Nucleus (SCN)

- The SCN is the "master clock" of our circadian (24-hour) biological rhythms.
- The SCN is very sensitive to light! For this reason, light at night can shift our rhythms to a later time.
- Light at night also has an alerting effect.

Melatonin

- Sometimes called "the hormone of the dark."
- Promotes sleepiness.
- Melatonin is secreted only in the absence of light and only at night. Light at night quickly suppresses melatonin.

(continued)

Light

- Interrupts the production of melatonin.
- Directly increases alertness.
- Interferes with winding down toward sleepiness.

"Even moderate light intensities, similar to indoor intensities, are able to cause substantial suppression of melatonin production" (Scheer & Czeisler, p. 5).

Darkness

- A powerful cue for reduced alertness and sleep.
- At night, darkness triggers a cascade of biological processes, including melatonin, which will help you fall asleep.
- Consider not turning on any major lights if you get up in the night (e.g., to use the restroom). Keeping the lights low will avoid the suppression of melatonin.

Did You Know?

- Computers, TV, and cellphones are sources of light and can interfere with your brain getting ready for sleep.
- Falling asleep with your bedroom light on can suppress melatonin all night long.
- Sleeping with the radio, music, or TV on can interrupt your sleep, making it lighter and more fragmented.

Activities before Sleep

- A high level of physical activity keeps you more alert. Winding down means slowing down!
- A high level of mental activity also keeps you more alert. The best activities before bed are those that don't require a lot of mental effort or problem solving.
- Finally, a high level of emotional engagement also makes us more alert and can interfere with sleepiness. Try to keep your most intense conversations and interactions—especially negative or stressful ones—for earlier in the evening.
- On the other hand, activities that you find relaxing in a physical, mental, and emotional sense will help you to "wind down" before sleep.

(continued)

- What are some examples of relaxing wind-down activities?
  - Gentle stretching exercises
  - A warm bath or shower
  - Reading, meditation, or prayer
  - Talking with a supportive person
  - Listening to music or watching TV are relaxing for some people, but avoid intense experiences!

Questions

- How much light do you get before bedtime?
- What kinds of activities do you do before bedtime?
- Can you think of ways to improve your bedtime routine? Think about physical, mental, and emotional dimensions to your bedtime routine. Let's note these on your worksheet.

Positive Conditioning

Positive conditioning means creating a set of physical, mental, and emotional conditions that allow your brain to fall asleep. Conditioning means establishing a routine that automatically cues your brain and body to expect that sleep is near. Here are some factors that contribute to positive conditioning in the presleep period.

- Cool, comfortable, and comforting environment.
- Devise a wind-down routine to increase physical, mental, and emotional relaxation.
- Electronic curfew: Commit to switching off your devices 30–60 minutes before bedtime.
- Not a time to think or process.
  - Try journaling or making to-do lists earlier in the evening rather than at bedtime.
  - Practicing relaxation skills for the mind and body are more appropriate bedtime activities.

My Wind-Down

Things to do during wind-down	Things to avoid during wind-down

Our Perception of Sleep

Estimating sleep accurately is an incredibly difficult, if not impossible, task. For example, most people have had the experience of intending to take a nap for just 10 minutes but then waking to discover that an hour has passed. It felt like just a few minutes. It's very difficult to tell how much time has passed during sleep.

It's not just the total amount of sleep we obtain that is difficult to estimate. Research has shown that reliably estimating the time taken to get to sleep is also difficult, because sleep is defined by the absence of memories. Your sleep diary is still very useful for planning and monitoring progress in treatment but the sleep diary gives us *estimates* of your sleep.

That is, it is very hard to remember exactly when you fell asleep or to estimate the time taken to fall asleep, even with the help of a clock. You might check the clock at 1:00 A.M. and then recheck it at 1:30 A.M. Between these two times, you might briefly fall asleep. A final reason that sleep estimation is difficult may be more surprising. We typically think of sleep and wakefulness as "all-or-nothing" phenomena, that is, that we must be either sleeping or awake. However, we now know from sophisticated EEG and brain imaging studies that sleep does not occur at the same time or with the same intensity in different parts of the brain. Thus, difficulties with sleep estimation may also reflect alterations in regional sleep.

Do you know the saying "Time flies when you're having fun"? The opposite also seems to be true. When you were a kid at school, do you remember knowing that there was 5 minutes until the bell rang signaling school is out? Yet in watching the clock, 5 minutes seemed to take forever. You weren't having fun and time crawled! Similarly, there is evidence that people who are tense and anxious in bed feel like more time has passed than actually has.

We also have difficulty with accurately determining the quality of our sleep. On waking, if we think, "I feel terrible. I must not have slept well," we are unlikely to be correct. We have to pass through the transition from sleep to wake, a state known as "sleep inertia." We often feel groggy, find it hard to get out of bed, and feel that if we were able to stay in bed we'd fall asleep again immediately. These feelings are normal and, fortunately, they pass quickly. They certainly do not reflect the quality of sleep obtained.

In fact, in the same way that our body automatically prompts us to breathe or to digest the food we eat, during sleep our body will automatically take the type and quality of sleep it needs. So if you have slept poorly for a few nights your body will recoup, immediately on nodding off, the type of sleep it most needs. That is, the human body keeps watch and looks after all your sleep processes by itself. The technical term for this is homeostasis.

To summarize:

- The total amount of time slept and the time taken to fall asleep are difficult to estimate.
- There is a distinction between how much sleep you *feel* you get and how much you *actually* get. Your feeling may not be accurate.
- The homeostatic processes within the body ensure that you get the type of sleep you need when you need it.

Thinking Traps

It is so easy to fall into the following thinking traps. Do any of these listed below look familiar?

Black-and-White Thinking

This involves viewing a problem or situation as all or nothing, as one extreme or another. This type of thinking is unrealistic because life is rarely completely hopeless or absolutely fantastic—it is usually somewhere in between.

Overgeneralization

This involves taking one experience and assuming that it applies to every similar situation, without recognizing the ways in which the situations may differ. For example, "I never sleep at night" is an example of overgeneralization. It is generalizing from one or more bad nights of sleep to *all* nights. This type of thinking is unhelpful. If something happened once, it does not necessarily mean it will keep happening in the future. The use of words such as always, never, or nothing are often clues that someone is overgeneralizing.

Personalization

Taking responsibility and blame for negative events for which you are not really responsible. An example of this type of thinking is feeling responsible if the company you work for is having major financial difficulties, even though you have always worked hard and have earned significant sums of money for the company.

Mistaking Feelings for Facts

This involves confusing feelings with reality. For example, a person may believe that because she *feels* hopeless that she actually *is* hopeless or that because he *feels* stupid, he *is* stupid.

Jumping to Negative Conclusions

This involves drawing negative conclusions from a situation when there is no evidence for this negative interpretation. For example, assuming that "there is no point in trying for regular bedtimes and wake times. I know it won't help" is an example of jumping to negative conclusions.

Catastrophizing

This involves assuming a situation has been or will be a complete and total disaster. For example, if you woke up on a Monday morning feeling tired and know the day will involve an important meeting at work, you think, "This is a disaster. I'm too tired to cope." Or "I'm ruined. I'm out of a job for sure." These are examples of catastrophizing.

Thinking traps such as those we've listed can have powerful effects on how we feel and on our self-confidence.

For Parents and Other Caregivers:
Your Role in Your Child's Sleep Coaching Experience

The growing science of behavior change suggests that there are two broad sources of motivation for teens to engage in healthier behaviors: the first are extrinsic sources of motivation, and the second are intrinsic motivation sources of motivation.

Extrinsic sources of motivation often involve external sources (e.g., pleasing or avoiding punishments from a parent, coach, or teacher). The external sources try to enforce or insist that the teen comply with or engage in a desired behavior. Enforcement can involve sanctions or threats. Extrinsic sources of motivation can contribute to teens feeling guilty, self-reproachful, pressured, tense, and anxious. The teen might engage with the desired behavior but does so because he or she feels obligated to and not because he or she wants to, and the behavior change is typically short term and not maintained.

Intrinsic sources of motivation often involves the teen identifying the value of a new behavior, seeing it as consistent with his or her own values and goals, and accepting full responsibility for engaging in the behavior. This source of behavior change arises from within the teen, so it is fully self-determined. It also is more likely to lead to lasting behavior change.

In each session with your teen we will encourage you to hand over, to your teen, full responsibility for his or her sleep. Typically you will be invited into the last 5 minutes of each session so your teen can summarize the major points we covered in the session and can request, if desired, your practical and/or emotional support for improving his or her sleep. We find that when we place responsibility on you, the parent, the approach often backfires and can create morning wake-up battles and difficulties in getting to school. In contrast, when responsibility for change is given to the teen, a shift often occurs whereby the teen feels proud to be trusted with such an important domain in his or her life. One very important role you can play is a subtle one; it is to contribute to an emotional sense of safety, positive emotions, and good associations at bedtime and wake-up time, being careful not to create noise and distractions if your teen wishes to go to bed earlier.

Having said all of that, we may need to work closely with you to dial shifting responsibility up or down, depending on the developmental phase of your teen. Also there are some additional things you can do to "cheerlead" for your teen.

- Ask your teen what he or she learned in each sleep coaching session.
- Ask your teen if your support is desired in achieving his or her goals. *Let your teen take the lead. It's far more effective for your teen to be motivated by his or her own goals than for you to be the "sleep cop" around bedtimes and wake times.*
- Try to keep bedrooms cool and dark with no distractions.
- As a parent, it is ideal if *you* can make an effort to go to bed at roughly the same time every night.
- Consider setting family rules about turning off devices with screens 30 minutes prior to bedtime. Parents need to follow the rules too!

(continued)

- Use low-light settings on devices at least 1 hour before bedtime, including in the bathroom, to avoid stimulating your brains with the "blue light" from devices.
- Help your teen with time management so that he or she can avoid stimulating activities, including doing homework, at least 60 minutes prior to bedtime. Avoiding exercise at least 2 hours before bedtime is important too.
- As best you can, make bedtime (and wake time) positive times of the day.
- Regular breakfast and dinner times, with dinner ideally occuring between 6:00 and 7:30 P.M. can help your teen get sleepy at an earlier time of the night.

My Sleep Diary

Instructions

Use the guide below to clarify what is being asked for by each item of the sleep diary.

For *date and day of the week,* write the date and day of the morning you are filling out the diary.

Circle "A.M." or "P.M.," whichever applies when you fill in each time. A.M. indicates the time period from midnight to noon. P.M. indicates the time period from noon to midnight. (Midnight = 12:00 A.M.; noon = 12:00 P.M.) Also, note the night for which you are filling out the diary.

1. **Please list the time and length of naps you took yesterday.** A nap is a time you slept during the day, whether in or out of bed, and whether on purpose or not. Count all the times you napped from when you first got out of bed in the morning until you got into bed again at night. *Also note in total, how long you napped yesterday.* Estimate the total amount of time you spent napping in hours and minutes.

2a. **How many drinks containing alcohol did you have yesterday?** Enter the number of alcoholic drinks you had. One drink is defined as one 12-ounce beer (can), 5 ounces of wine, or 1½ ounces of liquor (one shot).

2b. **What time was your last alcoholic drink?** If you had an alcoholic drink yesterday, enter the time of day in hours and minutes of your last drink. If you did not have a drink, write "N/A" (not applicable).

3a. **How many caffeinated drinks (coffee, tea, soda, energy drinks) did you have yesterday?** Enter the number of caffeinated drinks (coffee, tea, soda, energy drinks) you had. For coffee and tea, one drink = 6–8 ounces, while for caffeinated soda one drink = 12 ounces.

3b. **What time was your last caffeinated drink yesterday?** If you had a caffeinated drink, enter the time of day in hours and minutes of your last drink. If you did not have a caffeinated drink, write "N/A" (not applicable).

4. **What time did you get into bed last night?** Enter the time that you actually got into bed. This time may be earlier than the time you began "trying" to fall asleep, for instance, if you got into bed to watch TV.

5. **What time did you try to go to sleep?** Enter the time you began "trying" to fall asleep.

6. **How long did it take you to fall asleep?** Counting from the time you began trying to fall asleep, how long did it take you to fall asleep?

7. **How many times did you wake up, not counting your final awakening?** How many times do you think you woke up between the time you first fell asleep and your final awakening?

(continued)

8. **For how long did each awakening last?** Write down the amount of time you were awake after you woke up in the middle of the night. For example, if you woke up the first time for 20 minutes, write 20 minutes in the first space. If you woke up a second time for an hour and a half, write 1 hour 30 minutes in the second space. If you didn't wake up, just leave the space(s) blank. If you woke up more than three times, you can write down those times.

9. **What time was your final awakening?** Enter the last time you woke up in the morning without returning to sleep.

10. **What time did you get out of bed for the day?** What time did you get out of bed with no further attempt at sleeping? This may be later than your final awakening time (for example, you may have woken up at 6:35 A.M. but did not get out of bed to start your day until 8:20 A.M.).

11. **How would you rate the quality of your sleep last night?** Would you say your sleep was good or poor?

My Sleep Diary

	Example							
Date	1/9/17							
Day	Monday							
For which night's sleep?	Sunday							
1. Please list the time and length of naps you took yesterday.	11:30–11:45 P.M. 3–5 P.M.							
2a. How many drinks containing alcohol did you have yesterday?	2 drinks	drinks	drinks	drinks	drinks	drinks	drinks	drinks
2b. What time was your last alcoholic drink?	7:30 A.M. / (P.M.)	A.M. / P.M.	A.M. / P.M.	A.M. / P.M.	A.M. / P.M.	A.M. / P.M.	A.M. / P.M.	A.M. / P.M.
3a. How many caffeinated drinks (coffee, tea, soda, energy drinks) did you have yesterday?	3 drinks	drinks	drinks	drinks	drinks	drinks	drinks	drinks

(continued)

My Sleep Diary *(page 2 of 3)*

3b. What time was your last caffeinated drink?	*8:00* (A.M.) / P.M.	A.M. / P.M.	A.M. / P.M.	A.M. / P.M.	A.M. / P.M.	A.M. / P.M.	A.M. / P.M.
4. What time did you get into bed last night?	*12:45* (A.M.) / P.M.	A.M. / P.M.	A.M. / P.M.	A.M. / P.M.	A.M. / P.M.	A.M. / P.M.	A.M. / P.M.
5. What time did you try to go to sleep?	*1:15* (A.M.) / P.M.	A.M. / P.M.	A.M. / P.M.	A.M. / P.M.	A.M. / P.M.	A.M. / P.M.	A.M. / P.M.
6. How long did it take you to fall asleep?	___ hr(s) *30* min(s)	___ hr(s) ___ min(s)	___ hr(s) ___ min(s)	___ hr(s) ___ min(s)	___ hr(s) ___ min(s)	___ hr(s) ___ min(s)	___ hr(s) ___ min(s)
7. How many times did you wake up, not counting your final awakening?	*2* times	times	times	times	times	times	times
8. For how long did each awakening last?	1st awakening *30* hr(s) ___ min(s) / 2nd awakening *1* hr(s) *30* min(s) / 3rd awakening ___ hr(s) ___ min(s)	1st awakening ___ hr(s) ___ min(s) / 2nd awakening ___ hr(s) ___ min(s) / 3rd awakening ___ hr(s) ___ min(s)	1st awakening ___ hr(s) ___ min(s) / 2nd awakening ___ hr(s) ___ min(s) / 3rd awakening ___ hr(s) ___ min(s)	1st awakening ___ hr(s) ___ min(s) / 2nd awakening ___ hr(s) ___ min(s) / 3rd awakening ___ hr(s) ___ min(s)	1st awakening ___ hr(s) ___ min(s) / 2nd awakening ___ hr(s) ___ min(s) / 3rd awakening ___ hr(s) ___ min(s)	1st awakening ___ hr(s) ___ min(s) / 2nd awakening ___ hr(s) ___ min(s) / 3rd awakening ___ hr(s) ___ min(s)	1st awakening ___ hr(s) ___ min(s) / 2nd awakening ___ hr(s) ___ min(s) / 3rd awakening ___ hr(s) ___ min(s)

(continued)

My Sleep Diary *(page 3 of 3)*

9. What time was your final awakening?	7:45 (A.M.) / P.M.	A.M. / P.M.	A.M. / P.M.	A.M. / P.M.	A.M. / P.M.	A.M. / P.M.	A.M. / P.M.
10. What time did you get out of bed for the day?	7:45 (A.M.) / P.M.	A.M. / P.M.	A.M. / P.M.	A.M. / P.M.	A.M. / P.M.	A.M. / P.M.	A.M. / P.M.
11. How would you rate the quality of your sleep last night? 1 2 3 4 5 6 7 Poor Sleep Excellent Quality Sleep Quality	1 *(poor)*						

TO BE COMPLETED BY CLINICIAN

Time in Bed (TIB)	___ hrs ___ min	___ hrs ___ min	___ hrs ___ min	___ hrs ___ min	___ hrs ___ min	___ hrs ___ min	___ hrs ___ min
Total Sleep Time (TST)	___ hrs ___ min	___ hrs ___ min	___ hrs ___ min	___ hrs ___ min	___ hrs ___ min	___ hrs ___ min	___ hrs ___ min
Sleep Efficiency (SE)							
Midsleep Time (MST)							

Weekly Average Values

TIB:

TST:

SE:

MST:

Capturing Negative Automatic Thoughts

Using the form below, monitor your negative automatic thoughts related to sleep problems. Write down the situation (e.g., waking up, trying to fall asleep) the emotion you felt at that time (anxious, tired, etc.), and the thoughts you had related to the sleep problem (worried you won't get enough sleep, etc.).

Situation	Emotion	Automatic thoughts

Note. Based on J. Beck (1997).

Evaluating Negative Automatic Thoughts

The next time you catch yourself thinking a negative thought, use this tool to discover how the thought is affecting you and to disclose thoughts that might be more helpful to you. Note your negative thought related to sleeping, what activity you're doing, and emotions you're feeling.

Then, respond to the questions that follow.

Negative Thought:

Current Situation:

Current Emotions:

Evaluate Your Negative Thought

1. Is there an alternative way of thinking in this situation?

2. What is the evidence *for* my thought? What is the evidence *against* my thought?

3. What's the worst that could happen? How likely is it? Could I live through it?

(continued)

Note. Based on J. Beck (1997).

4. What's the best that could happen? How likely is it? What's the most realistic outcome?

5. What effect does thinking this thought have on me? Is my thought helpful?

6. What effect could changing my thought have on me?

7. If a good friend was in this situation, what would I tell that friend?

8. How important will this situation seem when I'm 80 years old?

Outcome: What are you thinking and feeling now?

References

Aloia, M. S., Arnedt, J. T., Riggs, R. L., Hecht, J., & Borrelli, B. (2004). Clinical management of poor adherence to CPAP: Motivational enhancement. *Behavioral Sleep Medicine*, 2(4), 205–222.

Aloia, M. S., Di Dio, L., Ilniczky, N., Perlis, M. L., Greenblatt, D. W., & Giles, D. E. (2001). Improving compliance with nasal CPAP and vigilance in older adults with OSAHS. *Sleep and Breathing*, 5(1), 13–21.

Aloia, M. S., Smith, K., Arnedt, J. T., Millman, R. P., Stanchina, M., Carlisle, C., . . . Borrelli, B. (2007). Brief behavioral therapies reduce early positive airway pressure discontinuation rates in sleep apnea syndrome: Preliminary findings. *Behavioral Sleep Medicine*, 5(2), 89–104.

Aloia, M. S., Stanchina, M., Arnedt, J. T., Malhotra, A., & Millman, R. P. (2005). Treatment adherence and outcomes in flexible vs standard continuous positive airway pressure therapy. *CHEST Journal*, 127(6), 2085–2093.

American Academy of Sleep Medicine. (2005). *International classification of sleep disorders (ICSD): Diagnostic and coding manual* (2nd ed.). Westchester, IL: Author.

American Academy of Sleep Medicine. (2014). *International classification of sleep disorders: Diagnostic and coding manual* (3rd ed.). Darien, IL: Author.

American Psychiatric Association. (2013). *Diagnostic and statistical manual of mental disorders* (5th ed.). Arlington, VA.: Author.

Andersson, G. (2009). Using the Internet to provide cognitive behaviour therapy. *Behaviour Research and Therapy*, 47(3), 175–180.

Barbini, B., Benedetti, F., Colombo, C., Dotoli, D., Bernasconi, A., Cigala-Fulgosi, M., . . . Smeraldi, E. (2005). Dark therapy for mania: A pilot study. *Bipolar Disorder*, 7, 98–101.

Barlow, D. H., Allen, L. B., & Choate, M. L. (2004). Toward a unified treatment for emotional disorders. *Behavior Therapy*, 35, 205–230.

Bartel, K., & Gradisar, M. (2017). New directions in the link between technology use and sleep in young people. In S. Nevšímalová & O. Bruni (Eds.), *Sleep disorders in children* (pp. 69–80). Cham, Switzerland: Springer International.

Bartlett, D. (2011a). Cognitive behavioral therapy to increase adherence to continuous positive airway: Model I. Psycho-education. In M. Perlis, M. Aloia, & B. Kuhn (Eds.), *Behavioral treatments for sleep disorders: A comprehensive primer of behavioral sleep medicine interventions* (pp. 211–214). London: Elsevier.

Bartlett, D. (2011b). Cognitive behavioral therapy to increase adherence to continuous positive airway: Model II. Modeling. In M. Perlis, M. Aloia, & B. Kuhn (Eds.), *Behavioral treatments for sleep disorders: A comprehensive primer of behavioral sleep medicine interventions* (pp. 215–222). London: Elsevier.

Beck, A. T. (1976). *Cognitive therapy and the emotional disorders.* Madison, CT: International Universities Press.

Beck, A. T., Rush, A. J., Shaw, B. F., & Every, G. (1979). *Cognitive therapy of depression.* New York: Guilford Press.

Beck, J. S. (2005). *Cognitive therapy for challenging problems: What to do when the basics don't work.* New York: Guilford Press.

Beck, J. S. (2011). *Cognitive therapy: Basics and beyond* (2nd ed.). New York: Guilford Press.

Bei, B., Wiley, J. F., Trinder, J., & Manber, R. (2016). Beyond the mean: A systematic review on the correlates of daily intraindividual variability of sleep/wake patterns. *Sleep Medicine Reviews, 28,* 104–120.

Benca, R. M., Obermeyer, W. H., Thisted, R. A., & Gillin, J. C. (1992). Sleep and psychiatric disorders: A meta-analysis. *Archives of General Psychiatry, 49,* 651–668; discussion 669–670.

Benedetti, F., Colombo, C., Barbini, B., Campori, E., & Smeraldi, E. (2001). Morning sunlight reduces length of hospitalization in bipolar depression. *Journal of Affective Disorders, 62,* 221–223.

Bennett-Levy, J., Butler, G., Fennell, M. J. V., Hackmann, A., Mueller, M., & Westbrook, D. (2004). *The Oxford handbook of behavioural experiments.* Oxford, UK: Oxford University Press.

Bentall, R. P., Rowse, G., Shryane, N., Kinderman, P., Howard, R., Blackwood, N., . . . Corcoran, R. (2009). The cognitive and affective structure of paranoid delusions: A transdiagnostic investigation of patients with schizophrenia spectrum disorders and depression. *Archives of General Psychiatry, 66,* 236–247.

Billiard, M., Dolenc, L., Aldaz, C., Ondze, B., & Besset, A. (1994). Hypersomnia associated with mood disorders: A new perspective. *Journal of Psychosomatic Research, 38*(Suppl. 1), 41–47.

Blunden, S., Gregory, A., & Crawford, M. (2013). Development of a Short Version of the Dysfunctional Beliefs about Sleep Questionnaire for Use with Children (DBAS-C10). *Journal of Sleep Disorders, 6,* 8–10.

Bootzin, R. R. (1972). Stimulus control treatment for insomnia. *Proceedings of the 80th Annual Convention of the American Psychological Association, 7,* 395–396.

Bootzin, R. R., Epstein, D., & Wood, J. M. (1991). Stimulus control instructions. In P. J. Hauri (Ed.), *Case studies in insomnia* (pp. 19–28). New York: Plenum Press.

Bootzin, R. R., & Stevens, S. J. (2005). Adolescents, substance abuse, and the treatment of insomnia and daytime sleepiness. *Clinical Psychology Review, 25,* 629–644.

Borbely, A., & Wirz-Justice, A. (1982). Sleep, sleep deprivation and depression. *Human Neurobiology, 1,* 205–210.

Borntrager, C., Chorpita, B., Higa-McMillan, C., & Weisz, J. (2009). Provider attitudes toward evidence-based practices: Are the concerns with the evidence or with the manuals? *Psychiatric Services, 60*(5), 677–681.

Breslau, N., Roth, T., Rosenthal, L., & Andreski, P. (1996). Sleep disturbance and psychiatric disorders: A longitudinal epidemiological study of young adults. *Biological Psychiatry, 39*, 411–418.

Brondel, L., Romer, M. A., Nougues, P. M., Touyarou, P., & Davenne, D. (2010). Acute partial sleep deprivation increases food intake in healthy men. *American Journal of Clinical Nutrition, 91*(6), 1550–1559.

Broomfield, N. M., & Espie, C. A. (2005). Towards a valid, reliable measure of sleep effort. *Journal of Sleep Research, 14*(4), 401–407.

Broström, A., Nilsen, P., Gardner, B., Johansson, P., Ulander, M., Fridlund, B., & Årestedt, K. (2014, April 27). Validation of the CPAP Habit Index–5: A tool to understand adherence to CPAP treatment in patients with obstructive sleep apnea. *Sleep Disorders*. Epub.

Brown, T. A., & Barlow, D. H. (1992). Comorbidity among anxiety disorders: Implications for treatment and DSM-IV. *Journal of Consulting and Clinical Psychology, 60*, 835–844.

Buysse, D. J. (2014). Sleep health: Can we define it? Does it matter? *Sleep. 37*(1), 9–17.

Buysse, D. J., Ancoli-Israel, S., Edinger, J. D., Lichstein, K. L., & Morin, C. M. (2006). Recommendations for a standard research assessment of insomnia. *Sleep: Journal of Sleep and Sleep Disorders Research, 29*(9), 1155–1173.

Buysse, D. J., Angst, J., Gamma, A., Ajdacic, V., Eich, D., & Rössler, W. (2008). Prevalence, course, and comorbidity of insomnia and depression in young adults. *Sleep. 31*(4), 473.

Buysse, D. J., Cheng, Y., Germain, A., Moul, D. E., Franzen, P. L., Fletcher, M., & Monk, T. H. (2010). Night-to-night sleep variability in older adults with and without chronic insomnia. *Sleep Medicine, 11*(1), 56–64.

Buysse, D. J., Germain, A., Douglas, M. E., Franzen, P. L., Brar, L. K., Fletcher, M. E., . . . Monk, T. H. (2011). Efficacy of brief behavioral treatment for chronic insomnia in older adults. *Archives of Internal Medicine, 171*, 887–895.

Buysse, D. J., Reynolds, C. F., Kupfer, D. J., Thorpy, M. J., Bixler, E., Manfredi, R., . . . et al. (1994). Clinical diagnoses in 216 insomnia patients using the International Classification of Sleep Disorders (ICSD), DSM-IV and ICD-10 categories: A report from the APA/NIMH DSM-IV Field Trial. *Sleep. 17*, 630–637.

Buysse, D. J., Yu, L., Moul, D. E., Germain, A., Stover, A., Dodds, N. E., . . . Pilkonis, P. A. (2010). Development and validation of patient-reported outcome measures for sleep disturbance and sleep-related impairments. *Sleep. 33*, 781–792.

Carney, C. E., Buysse, D. J., Ancoli-Israel, S., Edinger, J. D., Krystal, A. D., Lichstein, K. L., & Morin, C. M. (2012). The consensus sleep diary: Standardizing prospective sleep self-monitoring. *Sleep. 35*, 287–302.

Carney, C. E., & Waters, W. F. (2006). Effects of a structured problem-solving procedure on pre-sleep cognitive arousal in college students with insomnia. *Behavioral Sleep Medicine, 4*(1), 13–28.

Carskadon, M. A., & Dement, W. C. (2017). Normal human sleep: An overview. In M. H. Kryger, T. Roth, & W. C. Dement (Eds.), *Principles and practice of sleep medicine* (6th ed., pp. 15–24). Philadelphia: Elsevier.

Casagrande, S. S., Wang, Y., Anderson, C., & Gary, T. L. (2007). Have Americans increased their fruit and vegetable intake?: The trends between 1988 and 2002. *American Journal of Preventive Medicine, 32*(4), 257–263.

Casement, M. D., & Swanson, L. M. (2012). A meta-analysis of imagery rehearsal for post-trauma nightmares: Effects on nightmare frequency, sleep quality, and posttraumatic stress. *Clinical Psychology Review, 32*(6), 566–574.

Cassoff, J., Knäuper, B., Michaelsen, S., & Gruber, R. (2013). School-based sleep promotion programs: Effectiveness, feasibility and insights for future research. *Sleep Medicine Reviews, 17*(3), 207–214.

Chambless, D. L., & Hollon, S. D. (1998). Defining empirically supported theories. *Journal of Consulting and Clinical Psychology, 1*, 7–18.

Chennaoui, M., Arnal, P. J., Sauvet, F., & Léger, D. (2015). Sleep and exercise: A reciprocal issue? *Sleep Medicine Reviews, 20*, 59–72.

Chorpita, B. F., Park, A., Tsai, K., Korathu-Larson, P., Higa-McMillan, C. K., Nakamura, B. J., . . . Krull, J. (2015). Balancing effectiveness with responsiveness: Therapist satisfaction across different treatment designs in the Child STEPs randomized effectiveness trial. *Journal of Consulting and Clinical Psychology, 83*(4), 709.

Clark, A. L., Crabbe, S., Aziz, A., Reddy, P., & Greenstone, M. (2009). Use of a screening tool for detection of sleep-disordered breathing. *Journal of Laryngology and Otology, 123*, 746–749.

Clark, D. M. (1999). Anxiety disorders: Why they persist and how to treat them. *Behaviour Research and Therapy, 37*(Suppl. 1), S5–S27.

Clark, D. M. (2004). Developing new treatments: On the interplay between theories, experimental science and clinical innovation. *Behaviour Research and Therapy, 42*, 1089–1104.

Clark, D. M., Ehlers, A., Hackmann, A., McManus, F., Fennell, M., Grey, N., . . . Wild, J. (2006). Cognitive therapy versus exposure and applied relaxation in social phobia: A randomized controlled trial. *Journal of Consulting and Clinical Psychology, 74*, 568–578.

Clark, D. M., Salkovskis, P. M., Hackmann, A., Wells, A., Ludgate, J., & Gelder, M. (1999). Brief cognitive therapy for panic disorder: A randomized controlled trial. *Journal of Consulting and Clinical Psychology, 67*, 583–589.

Clarke, G., Harvey, A. G., McGlinchey, E., Hein, K., Gullion, C., Dickerson, J., & Leo, M. C. (2015). Cognitive-behavioral treatment of insomnia and depression in adolescents: A pilot randomized trial. *Behavior Research and Therapy, 69*, 111–118.

Colombo, C., Benedetti, F., Barbini, B., Campori, E., & Smeraldi, E. (1999). Rate of switch from depression into mania after therapeutic sleep deprivation in bipolar depression. *Psychiatry Research, 86*, 267–270.

Daley, M., Morin, C. M., LeBlanc, M., Gregoire, J.-P., & Savard, J. (2009). The economic burden of insomnia: Direct and indirect costs for individuals with insomnia syndrome, insomnia symptoms, and good sleepers. *Sleep. 32*(1), 55–64.

de Bruin, E. J., Oort, F. J., Bögels, S. M., & Meijer, A. M. (2014). Efficacy of internet and group-administered cognitive behavioral therapy for insomnia in adolescents: A pilot study. *Behavioral Sleep Medicine, 12*(3), 235–254.

de Shazer, S., & Dolan, Y. (2012). *More than miracles: The state of the art of solution-focused brief therapy*. New York: Routledge.

Drager, L. F., Togeiro, S. M., Polotsky, V. Y., & Lorenzi-Filho, G. (2013). Obstructive sleep apnea: A cardiometabolic risk in obesity and the metabolic syndrome. *Journal of the American College of Cardiology, 62*(7), 569–576.

Duckworth, A. L., Grant, H., Loew, B., Oettingen, G., & Gollwitzer, P. M. (2011). Self-regulation strategies improve self discipline in adolescents: Benefits of mental contrasting and implementation intentions. *Educational Psychology, 31*, 17–26.

Edinger, J. D., Bonnet, M. H., Bootzin, R. R., Doghramji, K., Dorsey, C. M., Espie, C. A., . . . Stepanski, E. J. (2004). Derivation of research diagnostic criteria for insomnia: Report of an American Academy of Sleep Medicine Work Group. *Sleep. 27*, 1567–1596.

Edinger, J. D., Means, M. K., Stechuchak, K. M., & Olsen, M. K. (2004). A pilot study of inexpensive sleep-assessment devices. *Behavioral Sleep Medicine, 2*(1), 41–49.

Edinger, J. D., Wohlgemuth, W. K., Radtke, R. A., Marsh, G. R., & Quillian, R. E. (2001). Does cognitive-behavioral insomnia therapy alter dysfunctional beliefs about sleep? *Sleep. 24*, 591–599.

Egan, S. J., Wade, T. D., & Shafran, R. (2011). Perfectionism as a transdiagnostic process: A clinical review. *Clinical Psychology Review, 31*, 203–212.

Ehlers, A., & Clark, D. M. (2000). A cognitive model of posttraumatic stress disorder. *Behaviour Research and Therapy, 38*, 319–345.

Ehlers, A., Clark, D. M., Hackmann, A., McManus, F., Fennell, M., Herbert, C., & Mayou, R. (2003). A randomized controlled trial of cognitive therapy, a self-help booklet, and repeated assessments as early interventions for posttraumatic stress disorder. *Archives of General Psychiatry, 60*, 1024–1032.

Ehlers, C. L., Frank, E., & Kupfer, D. J. (1988). Social zeitgebers and biological rhythms: A unified approach to understanding the etiology of depression. *Archives of General Psychiatry, 45*, 948–952.

Ellard, K. K., Fairholme, C. P., Boisseau, C. L., Farchione, T. J. & Barlow, D. H. (2010). Unified protocol for the transdiagnostic treatment of emotional disorders: Protocol development and initial outcome data. *Cognitive and Behavioral Practice, 17*, 88–101.

Erman, M. K., Stewart, D., & Einhorn, D. (2007). Validation of the ApneaLink™ for the screening of sleep apnea: A novel and simple single-channel recording device. *Journal of Clinical Sleep Medicine, 3*, 387–392.

Espie, C. A. (2002). Insomnia: Conceptual issues in the development, persistence, and treatment of sleep disorder in adults. *Annual Review of Psychology, 53*, 215–243.

Espie, C. A., Inglis, S., Harvey, L., & Tessier, S. (2000). Insomniacs' attributions: Psychometric properties of the Dysfunctional Beliefs and Attitudes about Sleep Scale and the Sleep Disturbance Questionnaire *Journal of Psychosomatic Research, 48*, 141–148.

Fairburn, C. G., Cooper, Z., Doll, H. A., O'Connor, M. E., Bohn, K., Hawker, D. M., . . . Palmer, R. L. (2009). Transdiagnostic cognitive-behavioral therapy for patients with eating disorders: A two-site trial with 60-week follow-up. *The American Journal of Psychiatry, 166*, 311.

Fairburn, C. G., Cooper, Z., & Shafran, R. (2003). Cognitive behaviour therapy for eating disorders: A "transdiagnostic" theory and treatment. *Behaviour Research and Therapy, 41*, 509–528.

Farney, R. J., Walker, B. S., Farney, R. M., Snow, G. L., & Walker, J. M. (2011). The STOP-Bang equivalent model and prediction of severity of obstructive sleep apnea: Relation to polysomnographic measurements of the apnea/hypopnea index. *Journal of Clinical Sleep Medicine, 7*(5), 459.

Ford, D. E., & Kamerow, D. B. (1989). Epidemiologic study of sleep disturbances and psychiatric disorders: An opportunity for prevention? *Journal of the American Medical Association, 262,* 1479–1484.

Frank, E. (2005). *Treating bipolar disorder: A clinician's guide to interpersonal and social rhythm therapy.* New York: Guilford Press.

Frank, E., Kupfer, D. J., Thase, M. E., Mallinger, A. G., Swartz, H. A., Fagiolini, A. M., . . . Monk, T. (2005). Two-year outcomes for interpersonal and social rhythm therapy in individuals with bipolar I disorder. *Archives of General Psychiatry, 62,* 996–1004.

Frank, E., Swartz, H. A., & Kupfer, D. J. (2000). Interpersonal and social rhythm therapy: Managing the chaos of bipolar disorder. *Biological Psychiatry, 48,* 593–604.

Freeman, D., Brugha, T., Meltzer, H., Jenkins, R., Stahl, D., & Bebbington, P. (2010). Persecutory ideation and insomnia: Findings from the second British National Survey of Psychiatric Morbidity. *Journal of Psychiatric Research, 44*(15), 1021–1026.

Freeman, D., Pugh, K., Vorontsova, N., & Southgate, L. (2009). Insomnia and paranoia. *Schizophrenia Research, 108*(1), 280–284.

Freeman, D., Stahl, D., McManus, S., Meltzer, H., Brugha, T., Wiles, N., & Bebbington, P. (2012). Insomnia, worry, anxiety and depression as predictors of the occurrence and persistence of paranoid thinking. *Social Psychiatry and Psychiatric Epidemiology, 47*(8), 1195–1203.

Freeman, D., Waite, F., Startup, H., Myers, E., Lister, R., McInerney, J., . . . Luengo-Fernandez, R. (2015). Efficacy of cognitive behavioural therapy for sleep improvement in patients with persistent delusions and hallucinations (BEST): A prospective, assessor-blind, randomised controlled pilot trial. *The Lancet, Psychiatry, 2*(1), 975–983.

Galla, B. M., & Duckworth, A. L. (2015). More than resisting temptation: Beneficial habits mediate the relationship between self-control and positive life outcomes. *Journal of Personality and Social Psychology, 109*(3), 508.

Germain, A., Shear, M. K., Hall, M., & Buysse, D. J. (2007). Effects of a brief behavioral treatment for PTSD-related sleep disturbances: A pilot study. *Behaviour Research and Therapy, 45,* 627–632.

Giglio, L. M., Magalhães, P., Andersen, M. L., Walz, J. C., Jakobson, L., & Kapczinski, F. (2010). Circadian preference in bipolar disorder. *Sleep and Breathing, 14,* 153–155.

Gollwitzer, P. M. (1999). Implementation intentions: Strong effects of simple plans. *American Psychologist, 54,* 493–503.

Gollwitzer, P. M., & Sheeran, P. (2006). Implementation intentions and goal achievement: A meta-analysis of effects and processes. *Advances in Experimental Social Psychology, 38,* 69–119.

Gradisar, M., Dohnt, H., Gardner, G., Paine, S., Starkey, K., Menne, A., . . . Weaver, E. (2011). A randomized controlled trial of cognitive-behavior therapy plus bright light therapy for adolescent delayed sleep phase disorder. *Sleep. 34*(12), 1671–1680.

Gradisar, M., Gardner, G., & Dohnt, H. (2011). Recent worldwide sleep patterns and problems during adolescence: A review and meta-analysis of age, region, and sleep. *Sleep Medicine, 12*(2), 110–118.

Gradisar, M., Smits, M. G., & Bjorvatn, B. (2014). Assessment and treatment of delayed sleep phase disorder in adolescents: Recent innovations and cautions. *Sleep Medicine Clinics, 9*(2), 199–210.

Gradisar, M., Wolfson, A. R., Harvey, A. G., Hale, L., Rosenberg, R., & Czeisler, C. A. (2013). The sleep and technology use of Americans: Findings from the National Sleep

Foundation's 2011 Sleep in America poll. *Journal of Clinical Sleep Medicine, 9*(12), 1291–1299.

Granholm, E., Holden, J., Link, P. C., McQuaid, J. R., & Jeste, D. V. (2013). Randomized controlled trial of cognitive behavioral social skills training for older consumers with schizophrenia: Defeatist performance attitudes and functional outcome. *The American Journal of Geriatric Psychiatry, 21*(3), 251–262.

Greenberger, D., & Padesky, C. A. (2016). *Mind over mood: Change how you feel by changing the way you think* (2nd ed.). New York: Guilford Press.

Greer, S. M., Goldstein, A. N., & Walker, M. P. (2013). The impact of sleep deprivation on food desire in the human brain. *Nature Communications, 4,* 2259.

Gregory, A. M., Cox, J., Crawford, M. R., Holland, J., & Harvey, A. G. (2009). Dysfunctional beliefs and attitudes about sleep in children. *Journal of Sleep Research, 18*(4), 422–426.

Gruber, J., Harvey, A. G., Wang, P. W., Brooks, J. O., 3rd, Thase, M. E., Sachs, G. S., & Ketter, T. A. (2009). Sleep functioning in relation to mood, function, and quality of life at entry to the Systematic Treatment Enhancement Program for Bipolar Disorder (STEP-BD). *Journal of Affective Disorders, 114,* 41–49.

Harkin, B., Webb, T. L., Chang, B. P., Prestwich, A., Conner, M., Kellar, I., . . . Sheeran, P. (2016). Does monitoring goal progress promote goal attainment?: A meta-analysis of the experimental evidence. *Psychological Bulletin, 142*(2), 198–229.

Harvey, A. G. (2008). Insomnia, psychiatric disorders, and the transdiagnostic perspective. *Current Directions in Psychological Science, 17,* 299–303.

Harvey, A. G. (2016). A transdiagnostic intervention for youth sleep and circadian problems. *Cognitive and Behavioral Practice, 23*(3), 341–355.

Harvey, A. G., Bélanger, L., Talbot, L., Eidelman, P., Beaulieu-Bonneau, S., Fortier-Brochu, E., . . . Morin, C. M. (2014). Comparative efficacy of behavior therapy, cognitive therapy and cognitive behavior therapy for insomnia: A randomized controlled trial. *Journal of Consulting and Clinical Psychology, 82,* 670–683.

Harvey, A. G., Clark, D. M., Ehlers, A., & Rapee, R. M. (2000). Social anxiety and self-impression: Cognitive preparation enhances the beneficial effects of video feedback following a stressful social task. *Behaviour Research and Therapy, 38,* 1183–1192.

Harvey, A. G., & Eidelman, P. (2011). Intervention to reduce unhelpful beliefs about sleep. In M. Perlis, M. Aloia, & B. Kuhn (Eds.), *Behavioral treatments for sleep disorders: A comprehensive primer of behavioral sleep medicine interventions* (pp. 71–78). London: Elsevier.

Harvey, A. G., & Farrell, C. (2003). The efficacy of a Pennebaker-like writing intervention for poor sleepers. *Behavioral Sleep Medicine, 1,* 115–124.

Harvey, A. G., Lee, J., Williams, J., Hollon, S. D., Walker, M. P., Thompson, M. A., & Smith, R. (2014). Improving outcome of psychosocial treatments by enhancing memory and learning. *Perspectives on Psychological Science, 9,* 161–179.

Harvey, A. G., Murray, G., Chandler, R. A., & Soehner, A. (2011). Sleep disturbance as transdiagnostic: Consideration of neurobiological mechanisms. *Clinical Psychology Review, 31,* 225–235.

Harvey, A. G., & Payne, S. (2002). The management of unwanted pre-sleep thoughts in insomnia: Distraction with imagery versus general distraction. *Behaviour Research and Therapy, 40,* 267–277.

Harvey, A. G., Schmidt, D. A., Scarna, A., Semler, C. N., & Goodwin, G. M. (2005).

Sleep-related functioning in euthymic patients with bipolar disorder, patients with insomnia, and subjects without sleep problems. *American Journal of Psychiatry, 162,* 50–57.

Harvey, A. G., Sharpley, A., Ree, M. J., Stinson, K., & Clark, D. M. (2007). An open trial of cognitive therapy for chronic insomnia. *Behaviour Research and Therapy, 45,* 2491–2501.

Harvey, A. G., Soehner, A. M., Kaplan, K. A., Hein, K., Lee, J., Kanady, J., . . . Buysse, D. J. (2015). Treating insomnia improves sleep, mood and functioning in bipolar disorder: A pilot randomized controlled trial. *Journal of Consulting and Clinical Psychology, 83*(3), 564–577.

Harvey, A. G., & Spielman, A. (2011). Insomnia: Diagnosis, assessment and outcomes. In M. H. Kryger, T. Roth, & W. C. Dement (Eds.), *Principles and practice of sleep medicine* (5th ed., pp. 838–849). St. Louis, MO: Saunders.

Harvey, A. G., & Talbot, L. S. (2011). Intervention to reduce misperception. In M. Perlis, M. Aloia, & B. Kuhn (Eds.), *Behavioral treatments for sleep disorders: A comprehensive primer of behavioral sleep medicine interventions* (pp. 91–96). London: Elsevier.

Harvey, A. G., & Tang, N. K. Y. (2012). (Mis)perception of sleep in insomnia: A puzzle and a resolution. *Psychological Bulletin, 138,* 77–101.

Harvey, A. G., Watkins, E., Mansell, W., & Shafran, R. (2004). *Cognitive behavioural processes across psychological disorders: A transdiagnostic approach to research and treatment.* Oxford, UK: Oxford University Press.

Heath, M., Sutherland, C., Bartel, K., Gradisar, M., Williamson, P., Lovato, N., & Micic, G. (2014). Does one hour of bright or short-wavelength filtered tablet screenlight have a meaningful effect on adolescents' pre-bedtime alertness, sleep, and daytime functioning? *Chronobiology International, 31*(4), 496–505.

Hillman, D. R., Murphy, A. S., & Pezzullo, L. (2006). The economic cost of sleep disorders. *Sleep. 29*(3), 299–305.

Hlastala, S. A., Kotler, J. S., McClellan, J. M., & McCauley, E. A. (2010). Interpersonal and social rhythm therapy for adolescents with bipolar disorder: Treatment development and results from an open trial. *Depression and Anxiety, 27,* 456–464.

Hysing, M., Pallesen, S., Stormark, K. M., Lundervold, A. J., & Sivertsen, B. (2013). Sleep patterns and insomnia among adolescents: A population-based study. *Journal of Sleep Research, 22*(5), 549–556.

Insel, T. R. (2009). Translating scientific opportunity into public health impact: A strategic plan for research on mental illness. *Archives of General Psychiatry, 66*(2), 128–133.

Irwin, M. R., Cole, J. C., & Nicassio, P. M. (2006). Comparative meta-analysis of behavioral interventions for insomnia and their efficacy in middle-aged adults and in older adults 55+ years of age. *Health Psychology, 25,* 3–14.

Jansson-Fröjmark, M., Harvey, A. G., Lundh, L. G., Norell-Clarke, A., & Linton, S. J. (2011). Psychometric properties of an insomnia-specific measure of worry: The anxiety and preoccupation about sleep questionnaire. *Cognitive Behaviour Therapy, 40*(1), 65–76.

Jenni, O., Achermann, P., & Carskadon, M. A. (2005). Homeostatic sleep regulation in adolescents. *Sleep. 28*(11), 1446–1454.

Johns, M. W. (1991). A new method for measuring daytime sleepiness: The Epworth sleepiness scale. *Sleep. 14,* 540–545.

Johnson, S. L. (2005). Mania and dysregulation in goal pursuit: A review. *Clinical Psychology Review, 25,* 241–262.

Kanady, J. C., & Harvey, A. G. (2015). Development and validation of the Sleep InertiaQuestionnaire (SIQ) and Assessment of Sleep Inertia in Analogue and Clinical Depression. *Cognitive Therapy and Research, 39*(5), 601–612.

Kaplan, K. A., Gruber, J., Eidelman, P., Talbot, L. S., & Harvey, A. G. (2011). Hypersomnia in inter-episode bipolar disorder: Does it have prognostic significance? *Journal of Affective Disorders, 132*(3), 438–444.

Kaplan, K. A., & Harvey, A. G. (2009). Hypersomnia across mood disorders: A review and synthesis. *Sleep Medicine Reviews, 13,* 275–285.

Kaplan, K. A., & Harvey, A. G. (2013). Behavioral treatment of insomnia in bipolar disorder. *American Journal of Psychiatry, 170*(7), 716–720.

Kaplan, K. A., Talavera, D., & Harvey, A. G. (2016). *Rise and shine: A treatment experiment testing a morning routine to decrease subjective sleep inertia in insomnia and bipolar disorder.* Manuscript submitted for publication.

Kazdin, A. E., & Blase, S. L. (2011). Rebooting psychotherapy research and practice to reduce the burden of mental illness. *Perspectives on Psychological Science, 6,* 21–37.

Kazdin, A. E., & Rabbitt, S. M. (2013). Novel models for delivering mental health services and reducing the burdens of mental illness. *Clinical Psychological Science, 1*(2), 170–191.

Kline, C. E. (2014). The bidirectional relationship between exercise and sleep implications for exercise adherence and sleep improvement. *American Journal of Lifestyle Medicine, 8*(6), 375–379.

Krakow, B., Hollifield, M., Johnston, L., Koss, M., Schrader, R., Warner, T. D., . . . Prince, H. (2001). Imagery rehearsal therapy for chronic nightmares in sexual assault survivors with posttraumatic stress disorder: A randomized controlled trial. *JAMA, 286,* 537–545.

Krupp, L. B., LaRocca, N. G., Muir-Nash, J., & Steinberg, A. D. (1989). The fatigue severity scale: Application to patients with multiple sclerosis and systemic lupus erythematosus. *Archives of Neurology, 46*(10), 1121–1123.

Kushida, C. A., Littner, M. R., Morgenthaler, T., Alessi, C. A., Bailey, D., Coleman, J., Jr., . . . Wise, M. (2005). Practice parameters for the indications for polysomnography and related procedures: An update for 2005. *Sleep. 28*(4), 499–521.

Kyle, S. D., Morgan, K., Spiegelhalder, K., & Espie, C. A. (2011). No pain, no gain: An exploratory within-subjects mixed-methods evaluation of the patient experience of sleep restriction therapy (SRT) for insomnia. *Sleep Medicine, 12,* 735–747.

Lichstein, K. L. (1988). Sleep compression treatment of an insomnoid. *Behavior Therapy, 19,* 625–632.

Lichstein, K. L., Durrence, H. H., Riedel, B. W., & Bayen, U. J. (2001). Primary versus secondary insomnia in older adults: Subjective sleep and daytime functioning. *Psychology and Aging, 16,* 264–271.

Lichstein, K. L., Durrence, H. H., Taylor, D. J., Bush, A. J., & Riedel, B. W. (2003). Quantitative criteria for insomnia. *Behaviour Research and Therapy, 41*(4), 427–445.

Littner, M., Hirshkowitz, M., Kramer, M., Kapen, S., Anderson, W. M., Bailey, D., . . . Woodson, B. T. (2003). Practice parameters for using polysomnography to evaluate insomnia: An update. *Sleep. 26,* 754–760.

Liu, X., Buysse, D. J., Gentzler, A. L., Kiss, E., Mayer, L., Kapornai, K., . . . Kovacs, M. (2007). Insomnia and hypersomnia associated with depressive phenomenology and comorbidity in childhood depression. *Sleep. 30*, 83–90.

Lloyd, H. (2008). More than miracles: The state of the art of solution-focused brief therapy by Steve de Shazer and Yvonne Dolan with Harry Korman, Terry Trepper, Eric McCollum and Insoo Kim Berg. *Journal of Family Therapy, 30*(1), 115–116.

Lovato, N., Gradisar, M., Short, M., Dohnt, H., & Micic, G. (2013). Delayed sleep phase disorder in an Australian school-based sample of adolescents. *Journal of Clinical Sleep Medicine, 9*(9), 939–944.

McMakin, D. L., Siegle, G. J., & Shirk, S. R. (2011). Positive affect stimulation and sustainment (PASS) module for depressed mood: A preliminary investigation of treatment-related effects. *Cognitive Therapy and Research, 35*, 217–226.

Means, M. K., & Edinger, J. D. (2011). Exposure therapy for claustrophobic reactions to continuous positive airway pressure. In M. Perlis, M. Aloia, & B. Kuhn (Eds.), *Behavioral treatments for sleep disorders: A comprehensive primer of behavioral sleep medicine interventions* (pp. 183–194). London: Elsevier.

Meltzer, L. J., Phillips, C., & Mindell, J. A. (2009). Clinical psychology training in sleep and sleep disorders. *Journal of Clinical Psychology, 65*(3), 305–318.

Miklowitz, D. J., Otto, M. W., Frank, E., Reilly-Harrington, N. A., Wisniewski, S. R., Kogan, J. N., . . . Sachs, G. S. (2007). Psychosocial treatments for bipolar depression: A 1-year randomized trial from the systematic treatment enhancement program. *Archives of General Psychiatry, 64*, 419–426.

Miller, W. R., & Rollnick, S. (2013). *Motivational interviewing: Helping people change* (3rd ed.). New York: Guilford Press.

Mistlberger, R. E., Antle, M. C., Glass, J. D., & Miller, J. D. (2000). Behavioral and serotonergic regulation of circadian rhythms. *Biological Rhythm Research, 31*, 240–283.

Morin, C. M. (1993). *Insomnia: Psychological assessment and management.* New York: Guilford Press.

Morin, C. M., Blais, F., & Savard, J. (2002). Are changes in beliefs and attitudes about sleep related to sleep improvements in the treatment of insomnia? *Behaviour Research and Therapy, 40*, 741–752.

Morin, C. M., Bootzin, R. R., Buysse, D. J., Edinger, J. D., Espie, C. A., & Lichstein, K. L. (2006). Psychological and behavioral treatment of insomnia: An update of recent evidence (1998–2004). *Sleep. 29*, 1396–1406.

Morin, C. M., Culbert, J. P., & Schwartz, S. M. (1994). Nonpharmacological interventions for insomnia: A meta-analysis of treatment efficacy. *American Journal of Psychiatry, 151*, 1172–1180.

Morin, C. M., & Espie, C. A. (2003). *Insomnia: A clinical guide to assessment and treatment.* New York: Kluwer Academic/Plenum Press.

Murtagh, D. R., & Greenwood, K. M. (1995). Identifying effective psychological treatments for insomnia: A meta-analysis. *Journal of Consulting and Clinical Psychology, 63*, 79–89.

Neitzert Semler, C., & Harvey, A. G. (2004). Monitoring for sleep-related threat: A pilot study of the Sleep Associated Monitoring Index (SAMI). *Psychosomatic Medicine, 66*, 242–250.

Neitzert Semler, C., & Harvey, A. G. (2005). Misperception of sleep can adversely affect daytime functioning in insomnia. *Behaviour Research and Therapy, 43*, 843–856.

Nigro, C. A., Dibur, E., Aimaretti, S., González, S., & Rhodius, E. (2011). Comparison of the automatic analysis versus the manual scoring from ApneaLink™ device for the diagnosis of obstructive sleep apnea syndrome. *Sleep and Breathing, 15,* 679–686.

Nofzinger, E. A., Thase, M. E., Reynolds, C. F., 3rd, Himmelhoch, J. M., Mallinger, A., Houck, P., & Kupfer, D. J. (1991). Hypersomnia in bipolar depression: A comparison with narcolepsy using the multiple sleep latency test. *American Journal of Psychiatry, 148,* 1177–1181.

Nolen-Hoeksema, S., & Watkins, E. R. (2011). A heuristic for developing transdiagnostic models of psychopathology explaining multifinality and divergent trajectories. *Perspectives on Psychological Science, 6,* 589–609.

Norton, P. J., & Philipp, L. M. (2008). Transdiagnostic approaches to the treatment of anxiety disorders: A quantitative review. *Psychotherapy: Theory, Research, Practice, Training, 45,* 214.

O'Connor Christian, S. L., & Aloia, M. (2011). Motivational enhancement therapy: Motivating adherence to positive airway pressure. In M. Perlis, M. Aloia, & B. Kuhn (Eds.), *Behavioral treatments for sleep disorders: A comprehensive primer of behavioral sleep medicine interventions* (pp. 169–182). London: Elsevier.

Oettingen, G., Mayer, D., Timur Sevincer, A., Stephens, E. J., Pak, H., & Hagenah, M. (2009). Mental contrasting and goal commitment: The mediating role of energization. *Personality and Social Psychology Bulletin, 35,* 608–622.

Okawa, M., Uchiyama, M., Ozaki, S., Shibui, K., & Ichikawa, H. (1998). Circadian rhythm sleep disorders in adolescents: Clinical trials of combined treatments based on chronobiology. *Psychiatry and Clinical Neurosciences, 52,* 483–490.

Oktay, B., Rice, T. B., Atwood, C. W., Passero, M., Gupta, N., Givelber, R., . . . Strollo, P. J. (2011). Evaluation of a single-channel portable monitor for the diagnosis of obstructive sleep apnea. *Journal of Clinical Sleep Medicine, 7,* 384–390.

Onken, L. S., Carroll, K. M., Shoham, V., Cuthbert, B. N., & Riddle, M. (2014). Re-envisioning clinical science: Unifying the discipline to improve the public health. *Clinical Psychological Science, 2*(1), 22–34.

Ozminkowski, R. J., Wang, S., & Walsh, J. K. (2007). The direct and indirect costs of untreated insomnia in adults in the United States. *Sleep. 30*(3), 263.

Paine, S., & Gradisar, M. (2011). A randomised controlled trial of cognitive-behaviour therapy for behavioural insomnia of childhood in school-aged children. *Behaviour Research and Therapy, 49*(6), 379–388.

Park, A. L., Tsai, K. H., Guan, K., Reding, M. E., Chorpita, B. F., & Weisz, J. R. (2016). Service use findings from the Child STEPs Effectiveness Trial: Additional support for modular designs. *Administration and Policy in Mental Health and Mental Health Services Research, 43*(1), 135–140.

Patel, S. R., & Hu, F. B. (2008). Short sleep duration and weight gain: A systematic review. *Obesity, 16*(3), 643–653.

Perlis, M., Smith, M., Jungquist, C., & Posner, D. (2005). *The cognitive-behavioral treatment of insomnia: A session by session guide* New York: Springer Verlag.

Qaseem, A., Kansagara, D., Forciea, M. A., Cooke, M., & Denberg, T. D. (2016). Management of chronic insomnia disorder in adults: A clinical practice guideline from the American College of Physicians. *Annals of Internal Medicine, 165*(2), 125–133.

Ragette, R., Wang, Y., Weinreich, G., & Teschler, H. (2010). Diagnostic performance of single airflow channel recording (ApneaLink) in home diagnosis of sleep apnea. *Sleep and Breathing, 14,* 109–114.

Ree, M., & Harvey, A. G. (2004). Insomnia. In J. Bennett-Levy, G. Butler, M. Fennell, A. Hackman, M. Mueller, & D. Westbrook (Eds.), *Oxford guide to behavioural experiments in cognitive therapy* (pp. 287–305). Oxford, UK: Oxford University Press.

Regestein, Q. R., & Monk, T. H. (1995). Delayed sleep phase syndrome: A review of its clinical aspects. *American Journal of Psychiatry, 152,* 602–608.

Reppert, S. M., & Weaver, D. R. (2002). Coordination of circadian timing in mammals. *Nature, 418,* 935–941.

Richards, D., Bartlett, D. J., Wong, K., Malouff, J., & Grunstein, R. R. (2007). Increased adherence to CPAP with a group cognitive behavioral treatment intervention: A randomized trial. *Sleep. 30*(5), 635.

Riley, C., Lee, M., Cooper, Z., Fairburn, C. G., & Shafran, R. A. (2007). Randomised controlled trial of cognitive-behaviour therapy for clinical perfectionism: A preliminary study. *Behaviour Research and Therapy, 45,* 2221–2231.

Roennebert, T., & Foster, R. G. (1997). Twilight times: Light and the circadian system. *Photochemistry and Photobiology, 66,* 549–561.

Roth, T., Jaeger, S., Jin, R., Kalsekar, A., Stang, P. E., & Kessler, R. C. (2006). Sleep problems, comorbid mental disorders, and role functioning in the National Comorbidity Survey replication. *Biological Psychiatry, 60*(12), 1364–1371.

Rubak, S., Sandbæk, A., Lauritzen, T., & Christensen, B. (2005). Motivational interviewing: A systematic review and meta-analysis. *British Journal of General Practice, 55*(513), 305–312.

Sack, R. L., Auckley, D., Carskadon, M. A., Wright, K. P. J., Vitiello, M. V., & Zhdanova, I. V. (2007). Circadian rhythm sleep disorders: Part II. Advanced sleep phase disorder, delayed sleep phase disorder, free-running disorder, and irregular sleep–wake rhythm: An American Academy of Sleep Medicine Review. *Sleep. 30,* 1484–1501.

Sack, R. L., Brandes, R. W., Kendall, A. R., & Lewy, A. J. (2000). Entrainment of free-running circadian rhythms by melatonin in blind people. *New England Journal of Medicine, 343*(15), 1070–1077.

Sack, R. L., & Lewy, A. J. (2001). Circadian rhythm sleep disorders: Lessons from the blind. *Sleep Medicine Reviews, 5*(3), 189–206.

Salkovskis, P. M. (2002). Empirically grounded clinical interventions: Cognitive-behavioural therapy progresses through a multi-dimensional approach to clinical science. *Behavioural and Cognitive Psychotherapy, 30,* 3–9.

Scheer, F. A., & Czeisler, C. A. (2005). Melatonin, sleep, and circadian rhythms. *Sleep Medicine Reviews, 9*(1), 5–9.

Schlarb, A., Liddle, C., & Hautzinger, M. (2010). JuSt-a multimodal program for treatment of insomnia in adolescents: A pilot study. *Nature and Science of Sleep. 3,* 13–20.

Semler, C. N., & Harvey, A. G. (2004). An investigation of monitoring for sleep-related threat in primary insomnia. *Behaviour Research and Therapy, 42,* 1403–1420.

Sit, D., Wisner, K. L., Hanusa, B. H., Stull, S., & Terman, M. (2007). Light therapy for bipolar disorder: A case series in women. *Bipolar Disorder, 9,* 918–927.

Sivertsen, B., Pallesen, S., Stormark, K. M., Bøe, T., Lundervold, A. J., & Hysing, M. (2013). Delayed sleep phase syndrome in adolescents: Prevalence and correlates in a large population based study. *BMC Public Health, 13*(1), 1163.

Smith, M. T., Perlis, M. L., Park, A., Smith, M. S., Pennington, J., Giles, D. E., & Buysse, D. J. (2002). Comparative meta-analysis of pharmacotherapy and behavior therapy for persistent insomnia. *American Journal of Psychiatry, 159,* 5–11.

Sorensen, J. L., Rawson, R. A., Guydish, J. E., & Zweben, J. E. (2003). *Drug abuse treatment through collaboration: Practice and research partnerships that work.* Washington, DC: American Psychological Association.

Spielman, A. J., & Anderson, M. W. (1999). The clinical interview and treatment planning as a guide to understanding the nature of insomnia: The CCNY insomnia interview. In S. Chokroverty (Ed.), *Sleep disorders medicine: Basic science, technical considerations, and clinical aspects* (2nd ed., pp. 385–426). Boston: Butterworth-Heinemann.

Spielman, A. J., Saskin, P., & Thorpy, M. J. (1987). Treatment of chronic insomnia by restriction of time in bed. *Sleep. 10,* 45–56.

Spielman, A. J., Yang, C. M., & Glovinsky, P. B. (2011). Sleep restriction therapy. In M. Perlis, M. Aloia, & B. Kuhn (Eds.), *Behavioral treatments for sleep disorders: A comprehensive primer of behavioral sleep medicine interventions* (pp. 9–20). London: Elsevier.

Stepanski, E. J., Zorick, F., Roehrs, T., Young, D., & Roth, T. (1988). Daytime alertness in patients with chronic insomnia compared with asymptomatic control subjects. *Sleep. 11,* 54–60.

Stepnowsky, C. J., Marler, M. R., & Ancoli-Israel, S. (2002). Determinants of nasal CPAP compliance. *Sleep Medicine, 3*(3), 239–247.

Sundararaman, R. (2009). *The U.S. mental health delivery system infrastructure: A primer.* Washington, DC: Congressional Research Service.

Tang, N. K. Y., & Harvey, A. G. (2004). Correcting distorted perception of sleep in insomnia: A novel behavioural experiment? *Behaviour Research and Therapy, 42,* 27–39.

Tang, N. K. Y., & Harvey, A. G. (2006). Altering misperception of sleep in insomnia: Behavioral experiment versus verbal feedback. *Journal of Consulting and Clinical Psychology, 74,* 767–776.

Tang, N. K. Y., Schmidt, D. E., & Harvey, A. G. (2007). Sleeping with the enemy: Clock monitoring in the maintenance of insomnia. *Journal of Behavior Therapy and Experimental Psychiatry, 48,* 40–55.

Taylor, D. J., Jenni, O. G., Acebo, C., & Carskadon, M. A. (2005). Sleep tendency during extended wakefulness: Insights into adolescent sleep regulation and behavior. *Journal of Sleep Research, 14,* 239–244.

Taylor, D. J., & Pruiksma, K. E. (2014). Cognitive and behavioural therapy for insomnia (CBT-I) in psychiatric populations: A systematic review. *International Review of Psychiatry, 26*(2), 205–213.

Teachman, B. A. (2014). No appointment necessary: Treating mental illness outside the therapist's office. *Perspectives on Psychological Science, 9*(1), 85–87.

Titov, N., Dear, B. F., Schwencke, G., Andrews, G., Johnston, L., Craske, M. G. & McEvoy, P. (2011). Transdiagnostic internet treatment for anxiety and depression: A randomised controlled trial. *Behaviour Research and Therapy, 49,* 441–452.

Waite, F., Myers, E., Harvey, A. G., Espie, C. A., Startup, H., Sheaves, B., & Freeman, D. (2015). Treating sleep problems in patients with schizophrenia. *Behavioural and Cognitive Psychotherapy,* 1–15.

Walters, A. S., LeBrocq, C., Dhar, A., Hening, W., Rosen, R., Allen, R. P., & Trenkwalder, C. (2003). Validation of the International Restless Legs Syndrome Study Group rating scale for restless legs syndrome. *Sleep Medicine, 4*(2), 121–132.

Watkins, E. R., Mullan, E., Wingrove, J., Rimes, K., Steiner, H., Bathurst, N., . . . Scott, J. (2011). Rumination-focused cognitive-behavioural therapy for residual depression: Phase II randomised controlled trial. *British Journal of Psychiatry, 199,* 317–322.

Wegner, D. M., Schneider, D. J., Carter, S. R., & White, T. L. (1987). Paradoxical effects of thought suppression. *Journal of Personality and Social Psychology, 53*, 5–13.

Weisz, J. R., Chorpita, B. F., Palinkas, L. A., Schoenwald, S. K., Miranda, J., Bearman, S. K., . . . Martin, J. (2012). Testing standard and modular designs for psychotherapy treating depression, anxiety, and conduct problems in youth: A randomized effectiveness trial. *Archives of General Psychiatry, 69*(3), 274.

Weisz, J. R., Ng, M. Y., & Bearman, S. K. (2014). Odd couple?: Reenvisioning the relation between science and practice in the dissemination-implementation era. *Clinical Psychological Science, 2*(1), 58–74.

Wells, A. (1997). *Cognitive therapy of anxiety disorders: A practice manual and conceptual guide*. West Sussex, UK: Wiley.

Wirz-Justice, A., Benedetti, F., & Terman, M. (2009). *Chronotherapeutics for affective disorders: A clinician's manual for light & wake therapy*. Basel: Karger.

Wood, A. M., Joseph, S., Lloyd, J., & Atkins, S. (2009). Gratitude influences sleep through the mechanism of pre-sleep cognitions. *Journal of Psychosomatic Research, 66*(1), 43–48.

Wu, J. Q., Appleman, E. R., Salazar, R. D., & Ong, J. C. (2015). Cognitive behavioral therapy for insomnia comorbid with psychiatric and medical conditions: A meta-analysis. *JAMA Internal Medicine, 175*(9), 1461–1472.

Yates, B. T. (2011). Delivery systems can determine therapy cost, and effectiveness, more than type of therapy. *Perspectives on Psychological Science, 6*(5), 498–502.

Yu, L., Buysse, D. J., Germain, A., & Moul, D. (2012). Development of short forms from the PROMIS sleep disturbance and sleep-related impairment item banks. *Behavioral Sleep Medicine, 10*, 6–24.

Index

Note: *f* following a page number indicates a figure; *t* indicates a table.